THE MODERN BOOK OF MASSAGE

FIVE-MINUTE VACATIONS AND SENSUOUS ESCAPES

THE MODERN BOOK OF MASSAGE

FIVE-MINUTE VACATIONS AND SENSUOUS ESCAPES

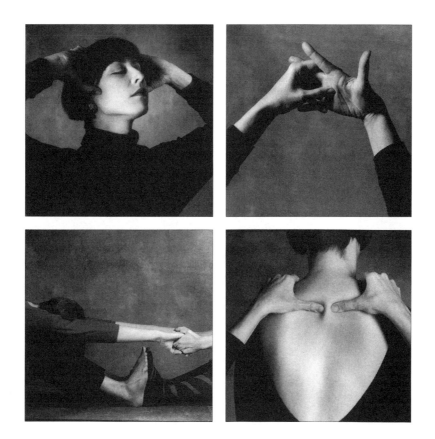

BY ANNE KENT RUSH • PHOTOGRAPHS BY PATRICK HARBRON

A BYRON PREISS/STONEWORK LTD. BOOK

A DELL TRADE PAPERBACK

A BYRON PREISS/STONEWORK LTD. BOOK

Published by Dell Publishing
a division of Bantam Doubleday Dell
Publishing Group, Inc.
1540 Broadway
New York, New York 10036

Library of Congress Cataloging-in-Publication Data
Rush, Anne Kent, 1945–
The modern book of massage: Five-minute vacations and sensuous escapes /
by Anne Kent Rush; photographs by Patrick Harbron.
p. cm.
"A Byron Preiss/Stonework Ltd. book."
ISBN 0-440-50545-3
1. Massage.   I. Title.
RA780.5.R873   1994
615.8'22–dc20   93-50206

Printed in the United States of America
Published simultaneously in Canada

October 1994
10 9 8 7 6 5 4

*This book
is dedicated to
The Dalai Lama of Tibet
and his work for peace.*

CONTENTS

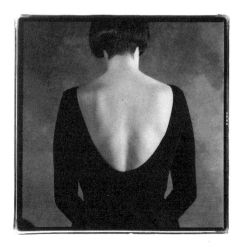

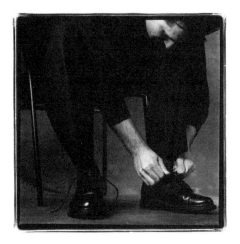

CONTENTS

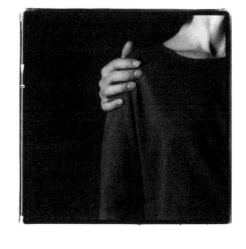

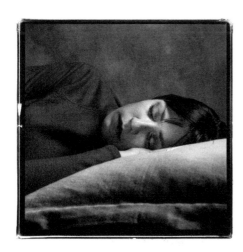

SECRETS OF LESS STRESS

This book offers a road map to exercise that can be done anytime, almost anywhere, and with or without a partner. Without leaving your home or office, you can use these techniques to equal the benefits of a weekend getaway. To learn to relax under pressure, you don't have to rent a car, fit into last year's bathing suit, worry about airline connections, or learn to speak Portuguese. If you are too busy for lengthy exercise or too tightly booked to take a Mediterranean cruise, relax. Medical science is on your side.

Two recent University of California–Berkeley studies present crucial facts about stress management in the Age of Overscheduling. Richard Lazarus and colleagues concluded that minor yet persistent annoyances have a more destructive effect on health than do grand-scale, isolated traumas. The good news is that little things mean a lot. Mini-vacations from your routine spaced throughout the day can produce significant stress reduction.

TAKING THE STRESS OUT OF STRESS MANAGEMENT

Scientific research now documents what we have long suspected: that living the good life is the best preventive medicine. Laughing bolsters your immune system and helps cure illness. Enjoying yourself slows down the aging process. Managing your stress levels improves the functioning of all your systems. Simple human touch can be more curative than cortisone.

A second U.C. Berkeley medical study uncovered a particularly noteworthy fact. To reduce stress, it's not sufficient to eliminate negative elements from your life. You need to add positive ones. To travel through life first class, focus on life's joys and increase your daily pleasures. Another expert in this department, Hedy Lamarr, sums up her approach to wellness in her autobiography, authoritatively titled *Ecstasy and Me*: "I don't fear anything I don't understand. When I start to think about it, I order a massage, and it goes away."

Advice worth trying. The exercises in this book are quick, sensual treats you can give yourself (or a friend) over the course of a day (or night). Of course, if you have more time, like Hedy, you could string them together in combinations of your choice to form a long massage. For basic maintenance, however, indulge in these body breaks one at a time throughout the day. They are five minute vacations to keep your compass pointing back to pleasure.

Bon voyage.

VACATION GUIDELINES

My most essential art is not the art of writing but...to change the worst into the not so bad. To lose and recover in the same instant that frivolous thing, a taste for life.
—Colette, **Looking Backward**

BODY POSTCARDS

Aches and pains are messages from your body about unfinished business. Stress-induced tension in an area of your body signifies suppression of the function of that part.

Release comes from performing the unfinished action comfortably. This is not to suggest that health demands that you express everything you feel without restraint. Other people's health is as important as your own. If your jaw and arm ache from a frustrating meeting, punching a co-worker is not the recommended relaxation. However, punching a pillow or a sports bag to complete the short-circuited action can help a lot.

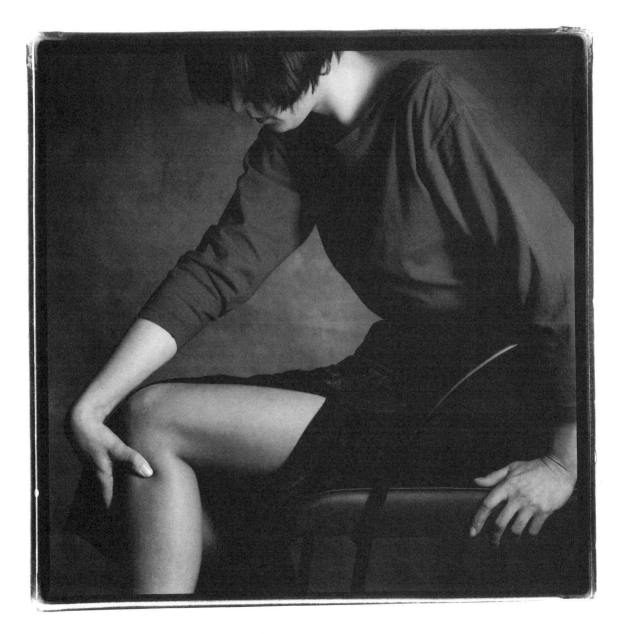

TOP SPOTS

No one knows why touch is so important.
—*Barbara Woodhouse,* **No Bad Dogs**

When the following treatments involve applying pressure on tension spots, acupressure charts are sometimes included, but they are only guidelines. Any spot that needs attention and feels better for being touched is the right spot to massage.

Trust your tactile sense to locate key spots. With practice you will become more and more sensitive to areas where blocked energy is concentrated and needs to be released throughout the body. Ask your friend if you are unsure of a point, and encourage him to let you know if he wants more or less pressure at any time.

At a high-energy spot you may feel a slight warmth and tingling. These sensations are caused by increased circulation of blood and body electricity. Improved circulation is a sign of relaxation. Visualizing this as you massage will intensify the healing process.

Work around an injury, not on top of it. Never press on an area that is bruised or damaged. Pain is a sign that the pressure is too hard or too fast. Lighten up immediately and press more slowly. Pain may add drama to a body treatment, but it leaves a residue of stress that is the opposite of relaxation and can cause new injuries. We need not punish ourselves for accumulating tension. For the fastest healing, apply pleasure.

Remember to stay relaxed while you massage. Lean rather than push to apply pressure. Alter your position anytime you feel uncomfortable. Mold your strokes to the shape of the muscles and define the bone structures. This increases the recipient's body awareness and sense of wholeness.

Daily Breath

Breathing techniques can be used by themselves or to improve the effectiveness of any exercise. Coordinating breathing with your movements will enhance circulation and increase healing. Holding your breath causes tension and restricts motion.

Inhale as you stretch out, and exhale as you curl in. Exhaling increases tension release. Allow your breathing to dictate when you begin a movement, rather than vice versa. Move smoothly and imagine that your breathing can massage your muscles from the inside.

In Focus

These are mental as well as physical vacations. To benefit most from your short breaks, stay focused on your body as you exercise. If your mind wanders to other activities or worries, you'll perform without increasing your awareness. The magic key to balance is attention. It's not so much what you do as how you do it that relaxes.

A Gift to Be Simple

The following exercises are quick and simple to perform, require no elaborate preparation, and can benefit the bodies of aspiring Olympic athletes and established couch potatoes alike. They are distillations of complex techniques that provide the user with the basics of body alignment. These are some that I have found to be the most effective in my twenty years' work in preventive health care. The most profound systems always appear simple.

One of the effects of doing these exercises is that you train your body to have new responses to pain and tension by substituting smooth movements for cramping. Relaxation becomes your reflexive response to stress. Trading pain for pleasure is a smart move. Feels good, too. Have fun.

This volume...placed upon the waistline and jerked up and down each morning... will reduce embonpoint and strengthen the abdominal muscles.

—*P. G. Wodehouse,* **The World of Jeeves**

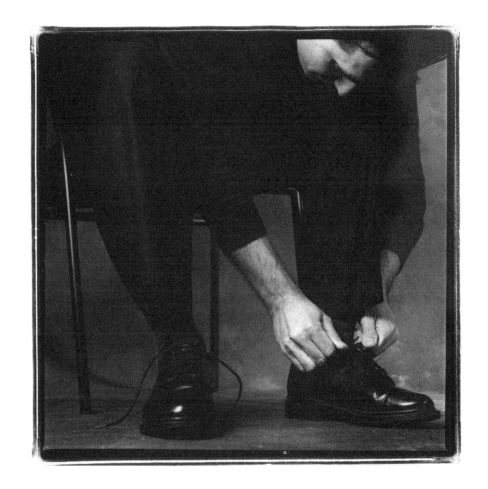

TAKE FIVE

UPPERS: FACE, NECK, AND SHOULDER ENERGIZERS

FOOT LIFTS

SPIRIT GUIDES:

LIFE AND BREATH

1

ENERGY TO GO

TAKE FIVE

The body has an endless longing to improve and to work.

—Marion Rosen, ***The Basic Back Book*** *by Anne Kent Rush*

What most of us call stress is in actuality too much of a very good thing. Stress is just an overbalance of energy for a situation, a sensory overload that makes us feel anxious instead of excited. We need the ability to regulate our energy levels, raising or lowering them to fit the needs of each situation. The techniques in this book enable you to do this in private and in public when you need to relax but can't exit. The exercises stimulate your circulation and ease tight muscles.

High stress nearly doubles your susceptibility to health problems. Luckily, laughter really is the best medicine. Enjoying yourself makes you less vulnerable to illness and injury. Simple steps like taking exercise breaks, sleeping enough, eating well, breathing deeply, and relaxing with friends all boost your levels of antibodies and disease-fighting cells. Energy comes from relaxing. No kidding.

Life is a daring adventure or nothing.

—Helen Keller, ***The Story of My Life***

Uppers: Face, Neck, and Shoulder Energizers

Enlightenment is not some good feeling or some particular state of mind. The state of mind that exists when you sit in the right posture is, itself, enlightenment.

—Suzuki Roshi, **Zen Mind, Beginner's Mind**

Facing the public in sit-down jobs, close-to-the-chest negotiations, or smile-intensive social occasions can tax your upper-body muscles. A stiff neck or a tight shoulder can lower your performance level and your mood. The following exercises release tension in these areas and revitalize your energy to face the rest of the day. A scalp, neck, and shoulder rub for a friend can be a luxurious treat.

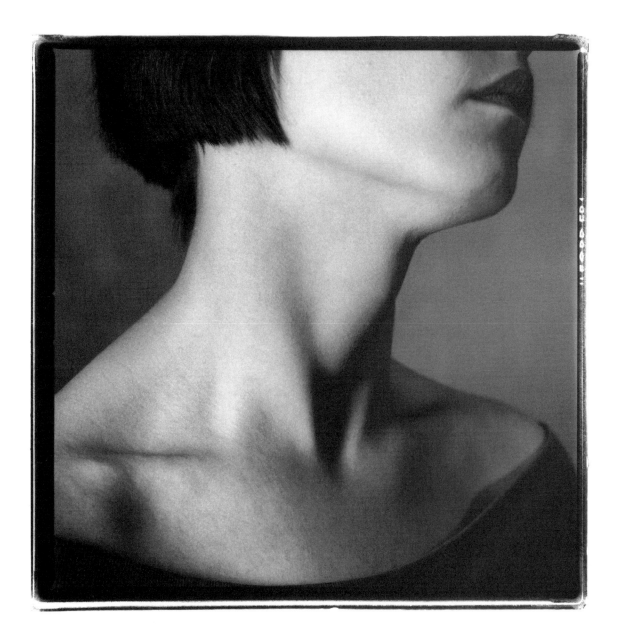

FACE POINTS

This chart shows some acupressure points on the face that help relax tension when massaged.

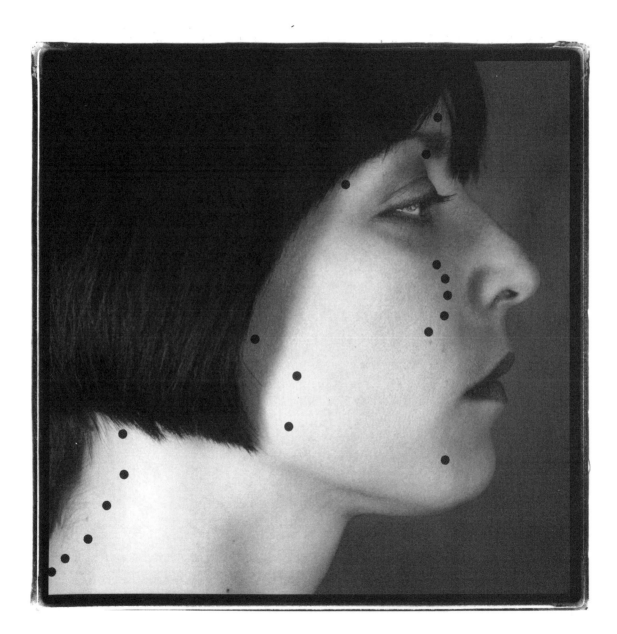

NECK FEATHERS

A stroke of relaxation.

1. Place fingertips lightly on cheekbones.

2. Draw them gently down either side of the neck.

3. Pull your fingertips lightly across the collarbone.

4. Speed up and press harder as you sweep across the tops of the shoulders and off. Then bring your hands back to the cheekbones to begin again.

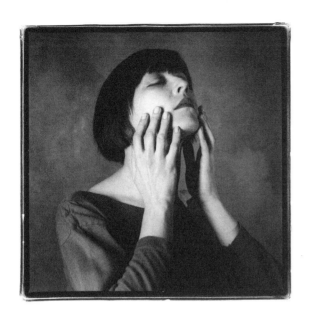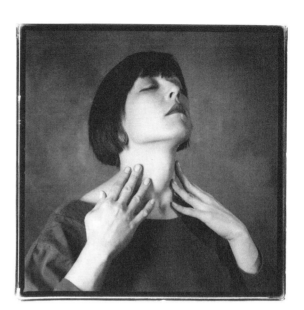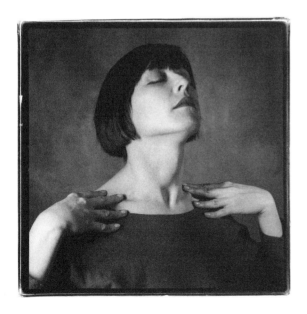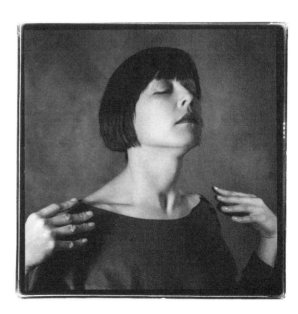

JAW RELAXER

To prevent coming unhinged.

1. Place your thumbs on the corners of your jaw hinges just in front of your earlobes, and your fingers on the back of your head. Gradually press into the jaw muscles with your thumbs.

2. Gradually release pressure and move to the next spot. Work from top of jaw bone down to the corners of your chin. We clench our jaws often during the day. Work here can be deeply relaxing for the whole face and neck.

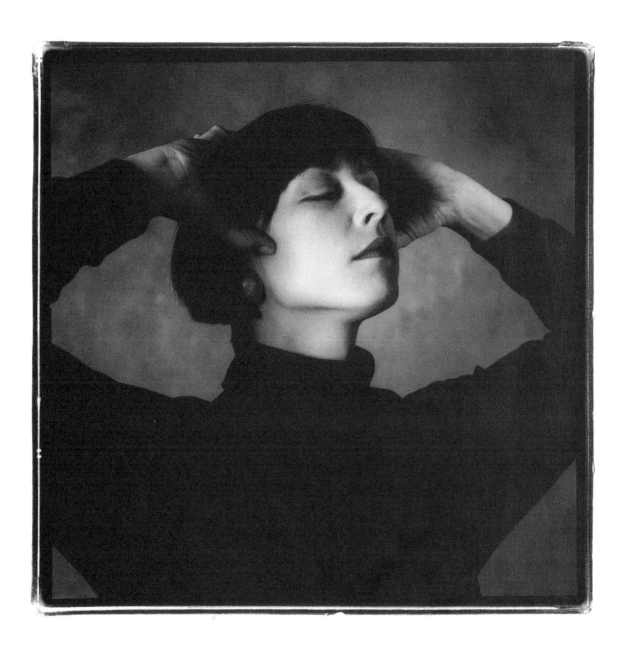

SINUS RELEASE

Fight pressure with pressure.

1. Place middle fingers under the cheekbones just to either side of the nose.

2. Apply gradual pressure. You can press quite deeply if it is comfortable.

3. Release the pressure as gradually as applied. This should quickly open your sinus area. Move your fingers to other spots along bony ridges here and repeat the sequence. Some spots will provide more release than others, depending on your condition each day.

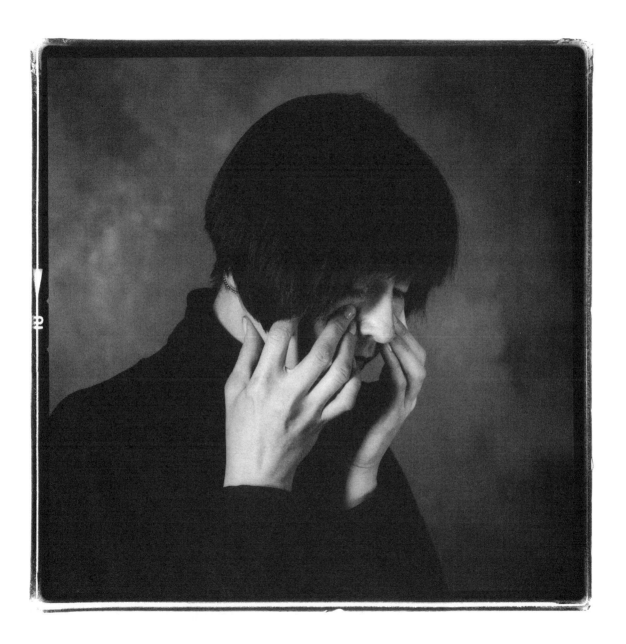

PUSH A HEAD

■

Brain-strain relief.

1. Make fists. Keep your thumbs free. Use the hard tips of your knuckles to apply pressure on the scalp just behind your temples. Then release.

2. Move your knuckles down just behind your ears onto the crescent-shaped mastoid bones. Press and release here, rocking from index fingers to baby fingers with the pressure while keeping your fists in place.

3. Find other tense areas on your scalp and use this fist-rocking pressure to relax them. Knuckles can be useful massage tools when your fingers are too tired to press hard.

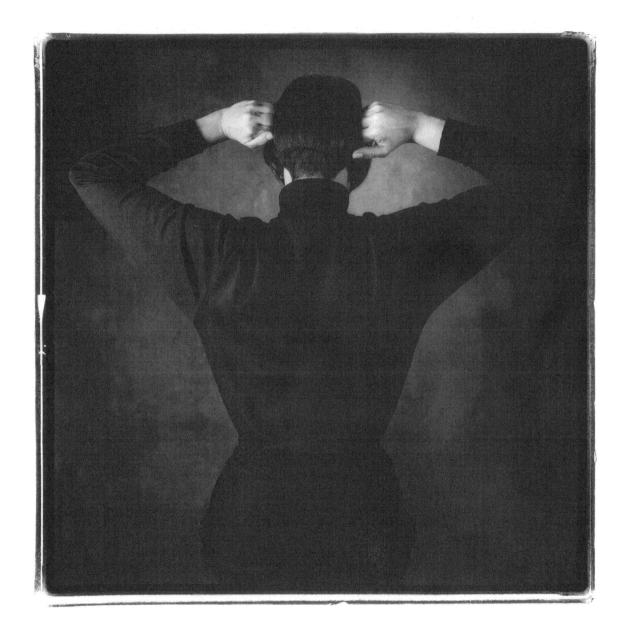

HEAD HAMMOCK

Imagine palm trees above you.

1. Clasp your hands behind your head and lean back.

2. Keeping your arms stationary, roll your resting head slowly from side to side as far as is comfortable. Try to give over the job of holding up your head to your hands so that you relax your neck and shoulder muscles and increase the scope of the turn.

3. Coordinate your breathing with the movement so that you inhale as you begin turning to one side and exhale as you turn the other way, to deepen the relaxation.

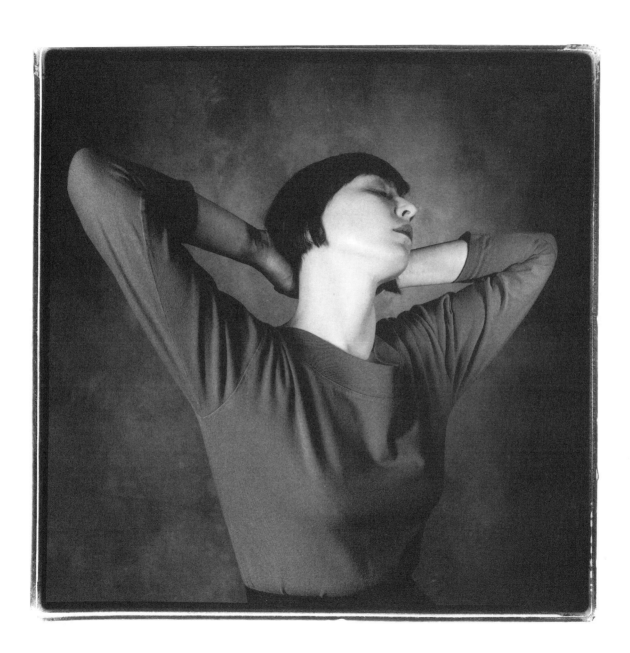

Neck and Shoulders

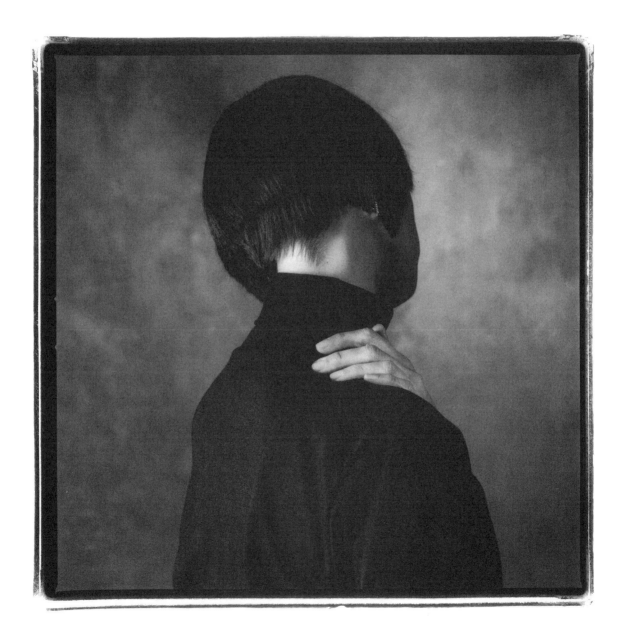

The Occipital Ridge

The indentation at the base of the skull where the neck begins, called the occipital ridge, contains a multitude of nerves that connect with key tension areas like the eyes, sinus, temples, forehead, neck, and shoulders. Massage on the points shown in the diagram can help release head, eye, sinus, and neck pains.

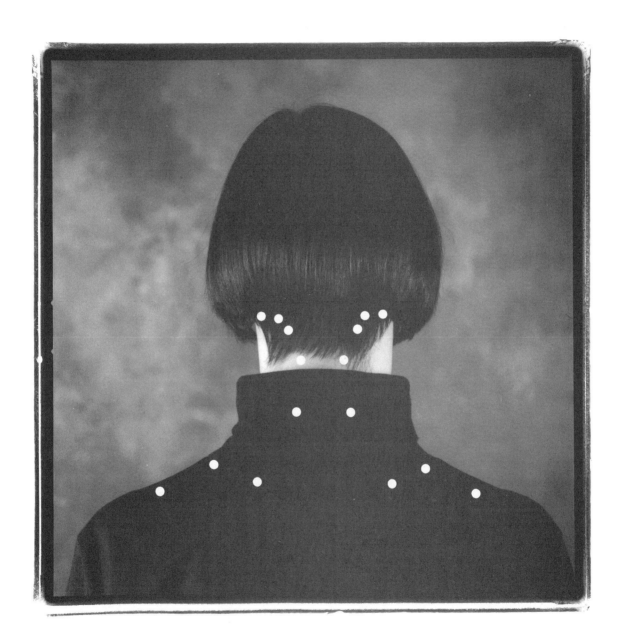

OCCIPUT PRESS

Release rigidity.

1. Tilt your head to the left and place your middle finger in the groove just to the right of the neck vertebrae at the base of the skull.

2. Press up into the groove. Gradually increase the pressure as you bring your head upright and your hand toward your neck.

3. When your hand is lodged in the crook of your neck securely, maintain this position and pressure. You can press more deeply as your neck muscles relax and any soreness there eases.

4. Release the pressure very gradually. Then repeat the massage on the left side of the neck with your left hand.

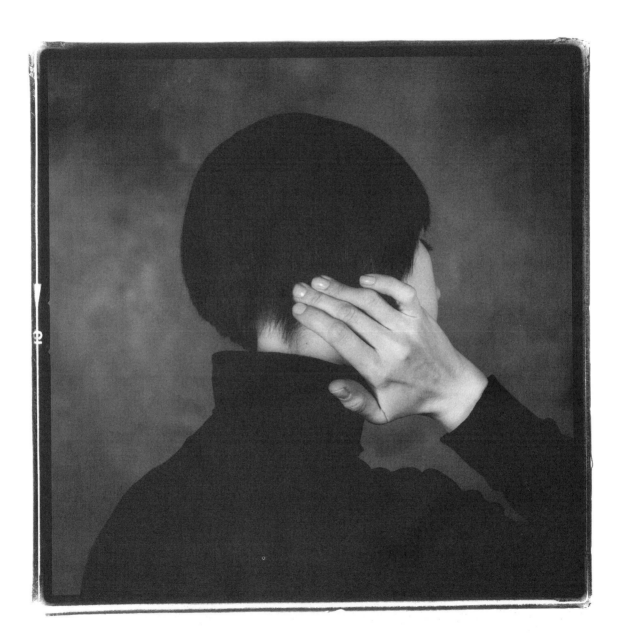

Neck and Shoulder Points

Very light pressure is applied to the front and sides of the neck. The back of the neck and shoulder points can tolerate deeper pressure with benefit. Massage along these points can relieve pain in the head, shoulders, and back.

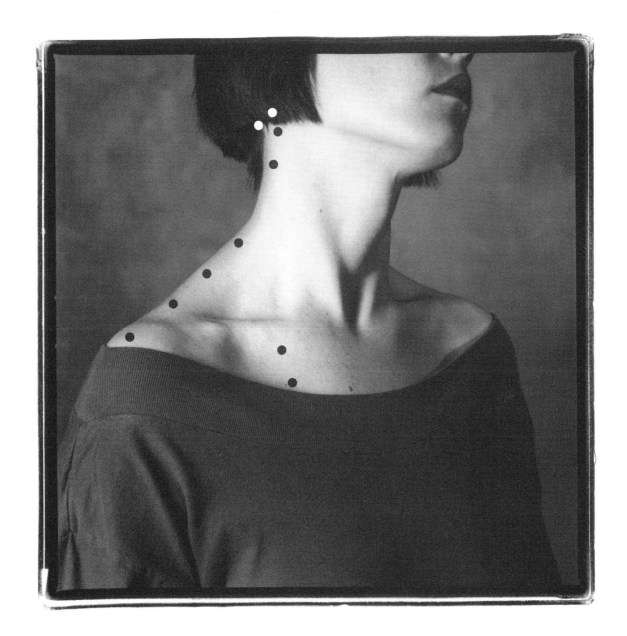

TRAPEZIUS POINTS

Send shoulder tension flying.

1. The trapezius muscles stretch from the side of the neck out to the tip of the shoulders and drape slightly onto the upper back. Most of us tense this area in response to daily pressures. Massage here can release much achiness and sense of burden or irritation.

2. Use your middle finger to apply gradual pressure on any sore spot along the muscle. Release as slowly as you apply pressure. A slow release enhances the feeling of uplift. Many headaches start from tight shoulder muscles. Work both shoulders.

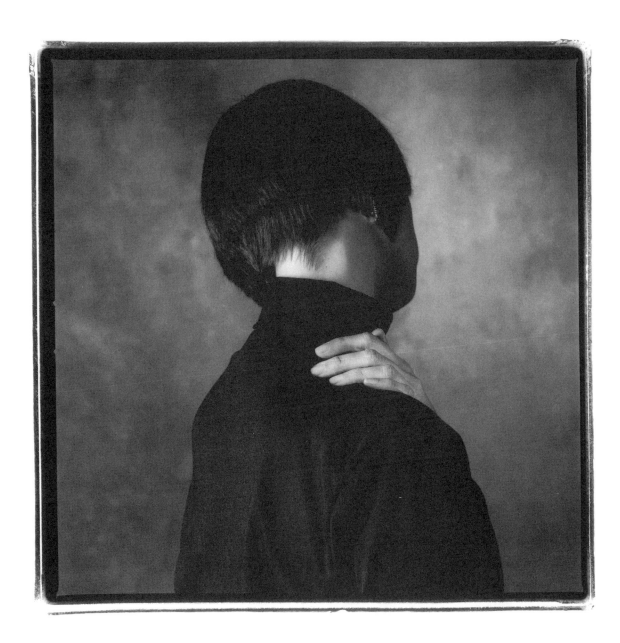

UPPER-BACK RELEASE

Ease a day's pain in the neck.

1. Lie on your back with your knees bent. Prop yourself up on your elbows, and allow your head to relax backward.

2. Relax your back and let your weight rest on your elbows. Release your neck muscles. With your neck relaxed, roll your head from side to side, aiming your chin toward your shoulders.

3. Bring your knees up over your chest and your forehead toward your knees for a final stretch. Exhale as you lower yourself to the floor.

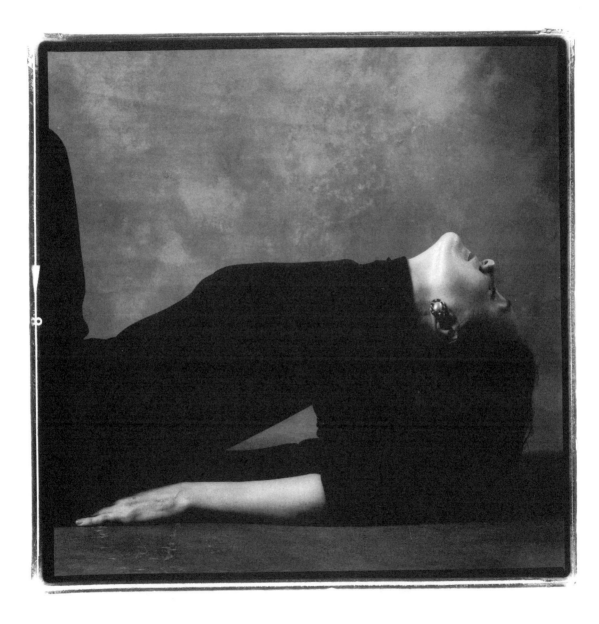

BLADE PROP

Shelve your shoulder tension.

1. Relax in a chair that reaches just above your shoulder blades at the back. Lift your shoulders and position the shoulder blades so they can rest on the top rung of the chair.

2. Gradually give over the work of holding up your back to the chair's edge as you release the tightness in your upper back and shoulders.

3. Lean forward and free your shoulders from the chair. Let your shoulders come down slowly.

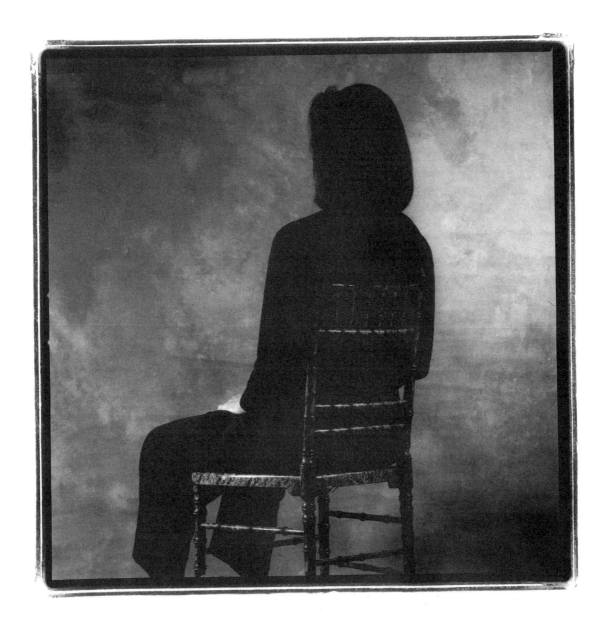

MIDDLE-BACK RELEASE

Movie-star stretch.

1. This can relax the hard-to-reach middle back and diaphragm. Clasp hands behind your head, spread your elbows back, and raise your chest to the fullest.

2. Inhale as you lean to the right, pointing your elbow toward the floor and raising the other elbow even higher. Be sure to stay upright rather than bend forward at the waist so that your ribs are stretched on the sides.

3. Exhale as you sit up and bring your head back to center. Repeat the stretch to the other side. Make the motion continuous from side to side, exhaling as you come back to center and inhaling as you stretch.

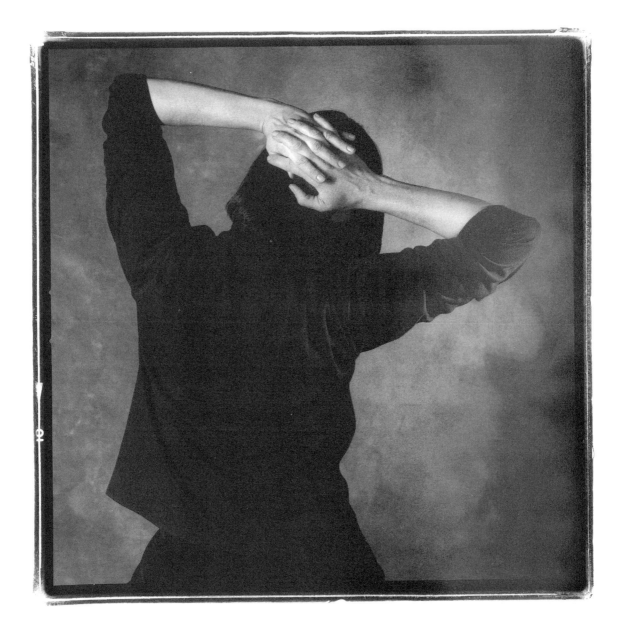

DESK REST

■■■■■

Spinal revival.

1. The curled position that a fetus rests in in the womb is one of the most relaxing positions for the body because the spine is not compressed and the arm, leg, and neck muscles are not stretched. Approximate the fetal curl while sitting to counteract the downward pressure on the body that builds when sitting a long time.

2. Rest your head on your arms on your desk. Raise the level of your knees to just above your hip joints by using a footstool or stacked books under your feet.

3. Close your eyes and breathe slowly and deeply. Even a minute or two will revive your eyes and spine.

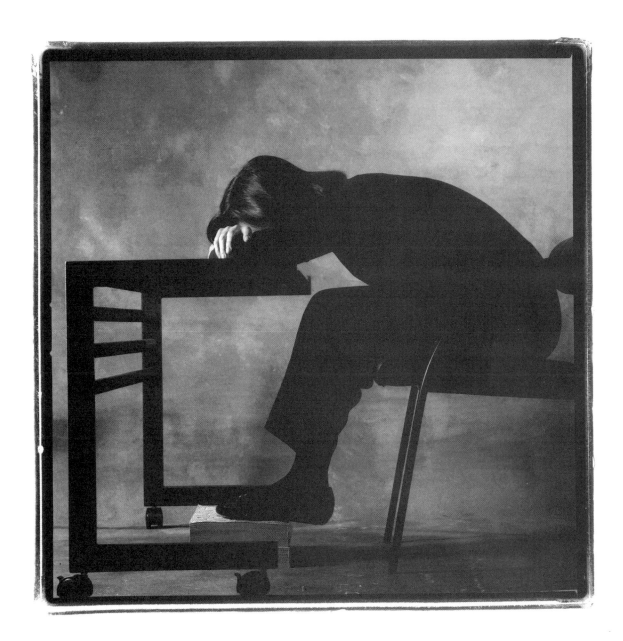

FOOT LIFTS

Put your feet in my lap and I will . . . ease the tightness of a long day.
—*Jeanette Winterson, **Written on the Body***

The feet psychologically represent our relationship to the earth, that is, to our roots, our mothers, our sense of solidity and reality. Physiologically, feet are an intense zone, because nerves from all over the body culminate there. Foot massage can send renewed energy to all parts of your body. When you feel like running away but have to stick around, a foot rub will help revive you to take a stand and like it. A foot massage for a friend is a gesture of support and acceptance.

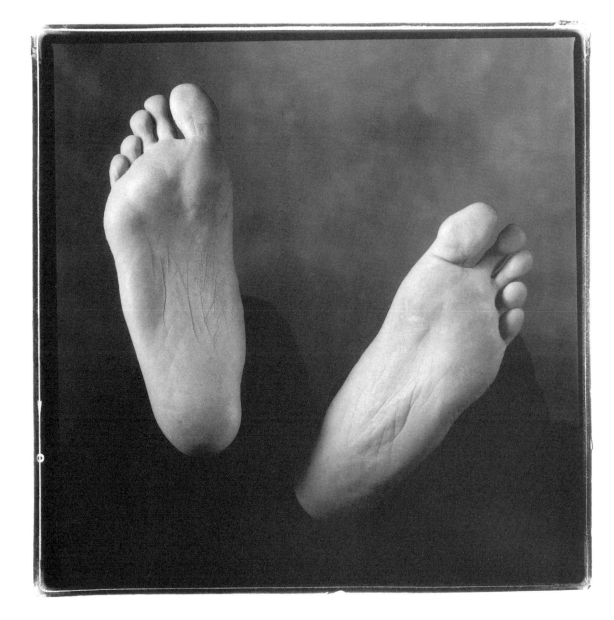

Foot Points

This chart shows the Oriental acupressure point system of areas to massage to help heal the corresponding organs and body parts.

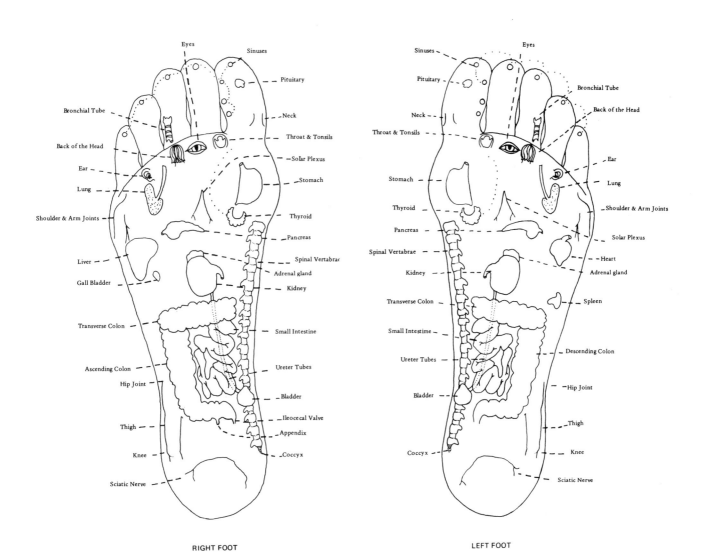

RIGHT FOOT

LEFT FOOT

STEP SLIDE

Arch march.

1. Slide your arches one after the other in close succession over the edge of a step or big book. Rounded steps feel best, but books work almost as well.

2. Vary the pace and pressure, and brace yourself on a desk or wall so you can really slide.

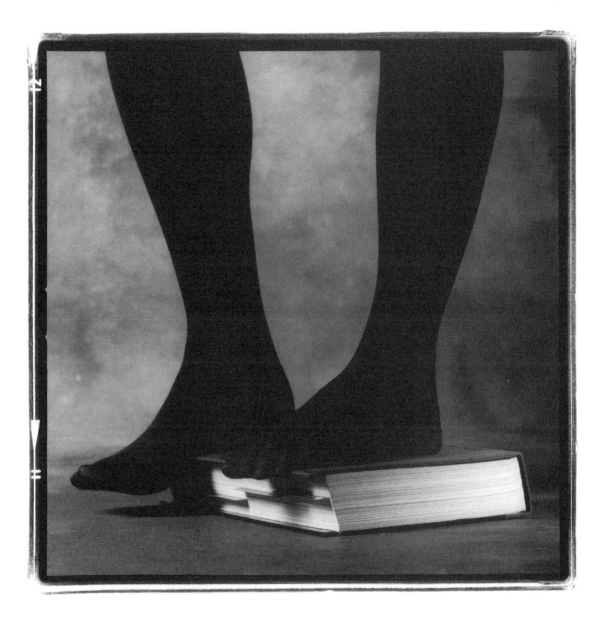

FOOT BALL

Sole roll.

1. A play ball can become a stimulating massage tool. Choose a solid rubber or plastic ball that fits in your arch comfortably.

2. While standing or sitting, lean onto the ball and roll it around the bottom of your foot. Change pressure as needed. Repeat on the other foot to refresh tired feet and tired spirits.

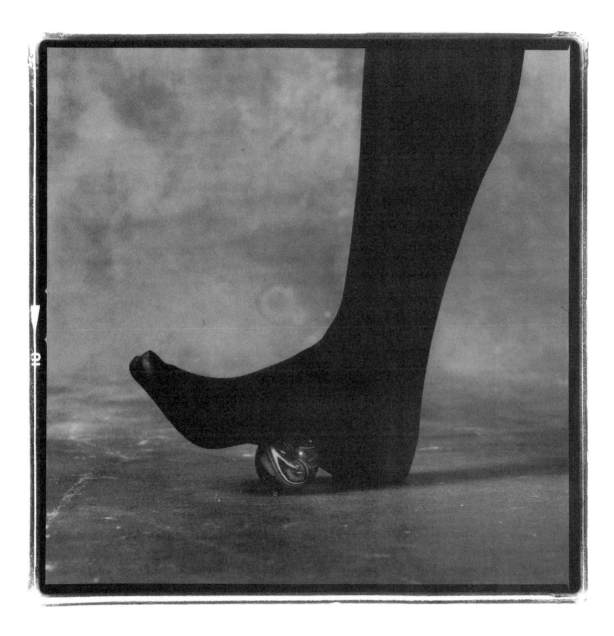

A R C H · P O I N T S   P R E S S

To the point.

1. The arch of the foot corresponds to the spine. Looking at the acupressure chart, press on the areas dotted on the chart along the arch.

2. Anywhere you find a tender spot, spend some extra time, because the corresponding body area is likely to be under stress and in need of revitalization.

3. You can reach many of the important arch points even with shoes on. Try this secret reviver under the table.

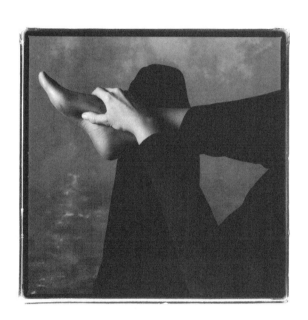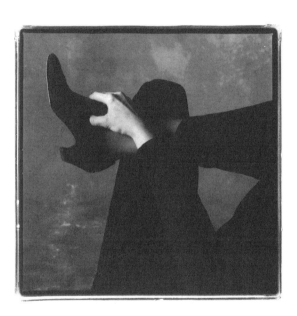

ANKLE-POINT PRESS

Ankle aches away.

1. Many spots around the ankle feel good to massage, but one under the ankle bone has particular relaxation punch. You can benefit from deep pressure here, so position your fingers so you can press hard with your thumb.

2. Under the ankle bone is a tiny tendon. Press under the tendon and lift up toward the ankle bone. Hold this lift and exert pressure. Start lightly and increase the pressure as any soreness there dissolves. Release very gradually.

3. Repeat on the other foot. This is a key acupuncture point that reaches many areas of the body. Hold the pressure as long as you can and you will be rewarded in tension release.

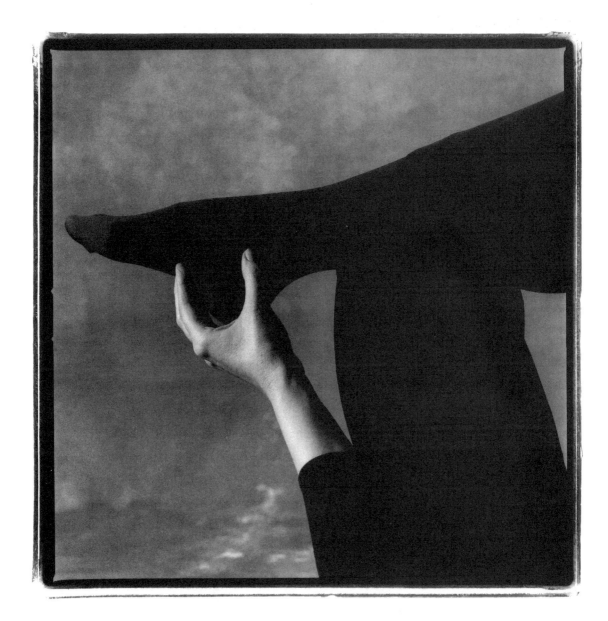

TENDON TUGS

Down in the valleys.

1. Keep your socks on unless you use oil or cream. The material provides a slippery surface for the massage. Find a groove between the bones of your foot and press in with your thumb.

2. Start as high up on the top of the foot as you like and drag your thumb all the way to the web between the toes. Deep pressure can be very relaxing. Explore all the grooves.

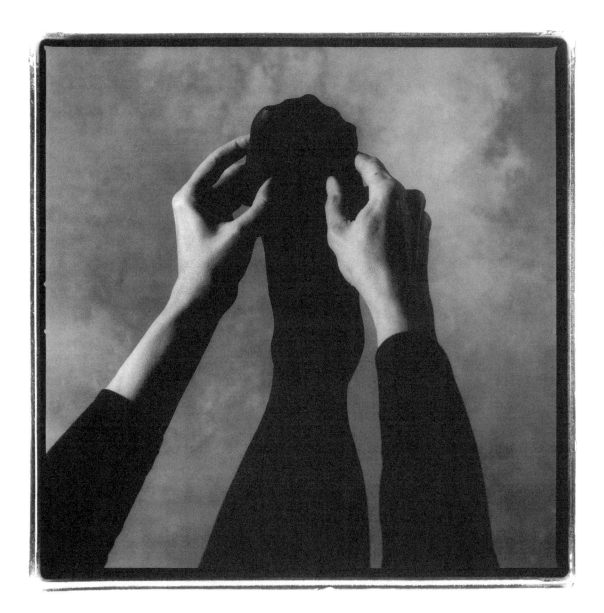

TOE FOLD

A gentle release.

1. This simple movement is quite relaxing when done slowly and gently. Place your fingertips at the base of the toes on the top of the foot. Gradually fold the toes down as far as is comfortable.

2. Release the stretch gradually. Then repeat on the other foot.

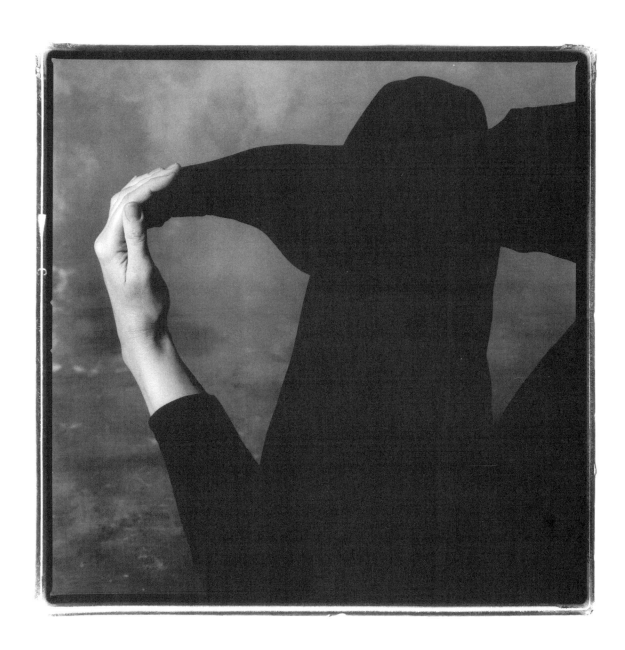

STACK AND STRETCH

Don't break; bend.

1. This is a good stretch for tense sitting muscles. Place one heel on top of the toes of the other foot and lean forward to grasp your toes.

2. Remain in this position long enough to: release your neck muscles so your chin comes toward your chest; release your back muscles so your spine forms a comfortable curve; and straighten out both legs as much as is possible. Lean forward at the waist and breathe deeply.

3. Release slowly. Repeat on the other foot.

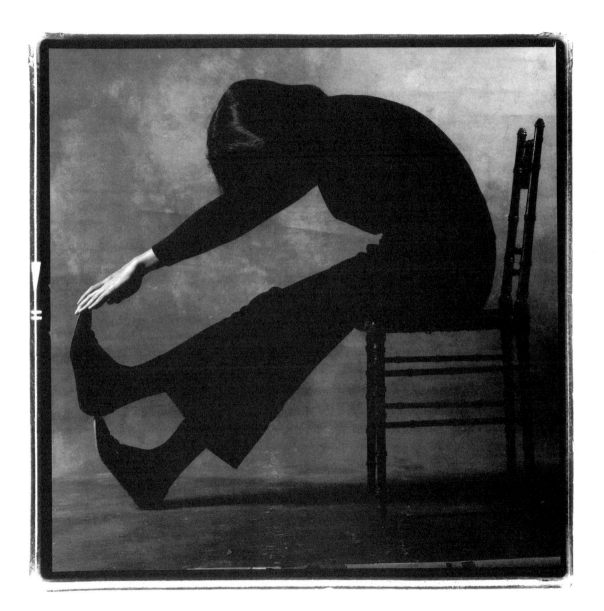

SPIRIT GUIDES

The part can never be well unless the whole is well.

—Plato, **Charmides,** c. 399 B.C.

Health is a state of complete physical, mental, and social
well-being and not merely the absence of disease or infirmity.

—**Constitution of the World Health Organization,** 1946

Any journey can be facilitated by a great guide. We have the ability to lead ourselves on inner explorations by mental role playing called visualization. During a quiet moment alone, close your eyes and relax your breathing. Imagine anyone you choose is guiding you through a spiritual quest. You can speak out loud to describe the events or simply allow images to appear. Let your mind form ideal pictures of where and how you'd like to be. These images are practice runs for acting on your highest concepts during your daily life and can help you define your direction when you are feeling lost or undecided.

The mind is part of the body, and balanced interaction between these aspects of ourselves maintains good health. Mental relaxation exercises round out our fitness regimes and can become our invisible weapons against stress during crisis. Even brief visualizations of places and people you love or images of your body's systems functioning well can help heal you and brighten your outlook. Invent and practice your own healing visions. They will bring positive results. Using images from your dreams or combining breathing exercises with visualization can be especially powerful. Breathing low in your body deepens the relaxation of your imagery exercises.

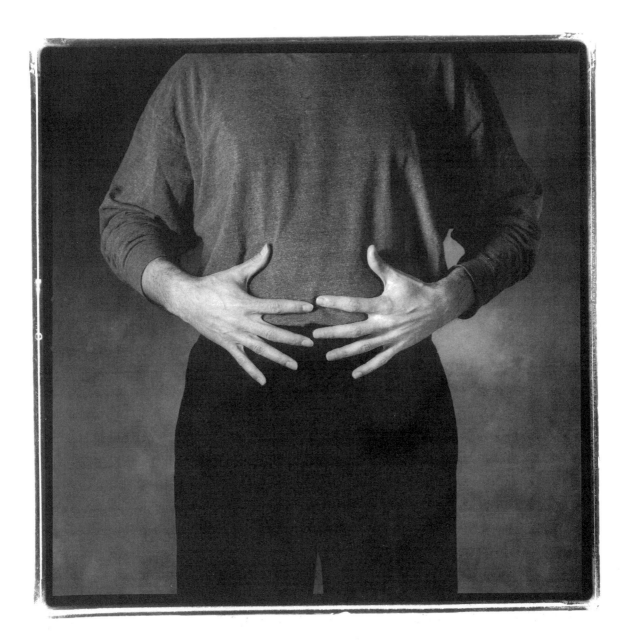

LIFE AND BREATH

All things share the same breath.

—*Chief Sealth, Duwamish Tribe,* **Seven Arrows** *by Hyemeyohsts Storm*

As you inhale, oxygen is drawn from the air around you into your lungs. In the exercises that follow, you'll be asked to visualize that you can breathe into a body part to relax it. This is not far from what really happens. From the lungs, oxygen is transferred to your blood cells, which carry it all over the body, where it is absorbed into your tissues. Oxygen uniting with tissue matter produces heat and keeps your body at a uniform temperature, which is why you can warm up your body by deep breathing. The improved circulation is relaxing and rejuvenating.

Oxygen deprivation can have serious consequences. You can live without food or water for many days, but you can only live without oxygen for about five minutes. Even relatively minor diminution of oxygen impairs vision, motor coordination, thought, judgment, and consciousness. These crucial aspects of our functioning are all affected by the level of oxygen reaching the body's key organs.

Fatigue, smoking, and chemical depressants such as alcohol all reduce the oxygen diffusion rate to the blood and thus impair judgment, mood, and performance. The reverse also applies. Improve your oxygen supply and you become more coordinated, more rational, more alert, and calmer.

The basic breathing exercises described here offer you methods for deepening your breathing, increasing your oxygen absorption, counteracting fatigue, reducing tension-induced anxiety, and lifting your mood. A deep breath anytime, anywhere, is one of your best body vacations. Sigh.

BELLY BREATH—SLOW

Treasures of the deep.

1. Breathing high in your chest is associated with fast-paced activity and agitation. Breathing deeper in your belly produces a sense of relaxation and calmness.

2. Anywhere you touch, your breathing will follow. Place your palms on your belly to help bring your breath there. Feel your abdomen rise as you inhale and sink down as you exhale.

3. Use slow belly breathing to restore calmness any time you feel too tense.

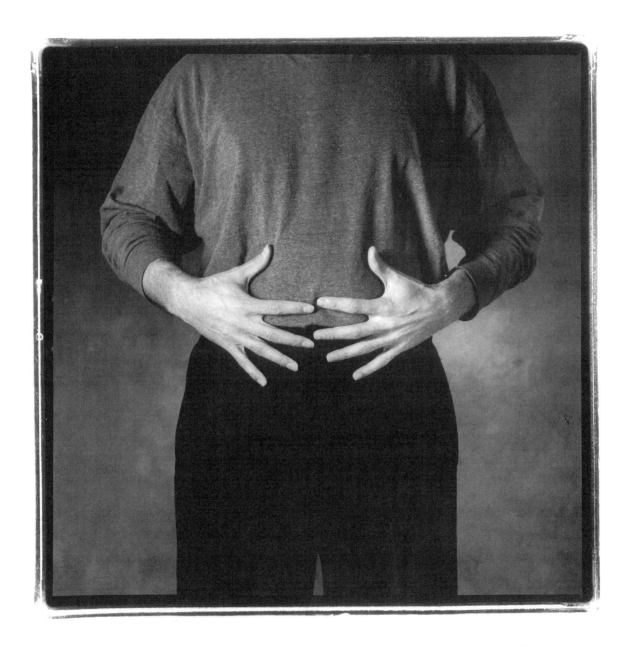

BELLY BREATH—FAST

Low blow.

1. This breath will bring you more energy. It should be done while you are sitting down, because sometimes it causes light-headedness.

2. Place your palms on your lower abdomen. Sit upright with a relaxed belly. Begin exhaling fast and deeply, speeding up the pace and depth as you go. Emphasize the exhalation pressure as you pull your belly muscles in.

3. If you feel light-headed, take a few slow breaths. Resume the fast exhalations when your head clears. Repeat whenever you feel drowsy.

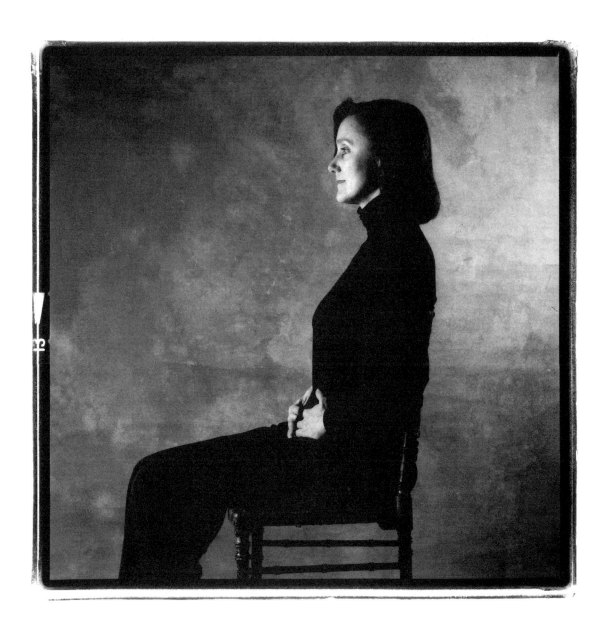

BREATHING INTO BODY PARTS

Spirit ball.

1. Try this technique with your hands and then with other areas. As you breathe, oxygen is drawn into your body and sent to various parts of your system through your bloodstream. Visualize this process and imagine you can direct the flow of oxygen to a specific body part.

2. Imagine you can send oxygen as you exhale down through your arms and into your hands. When you sense some warmth in your palms, bring your palms to face each other in front of your waist. The increased blood and electricity flow to the area can take on a shape, often a ball. Let your hands move around the energy shape, experimenting with how far apart or close to move them for the most intense sensation.

3. This exercise releases tension in the arms and hands. Try it before giving a massage to enhance the relaxation. Breathe into any body part you want to heal.

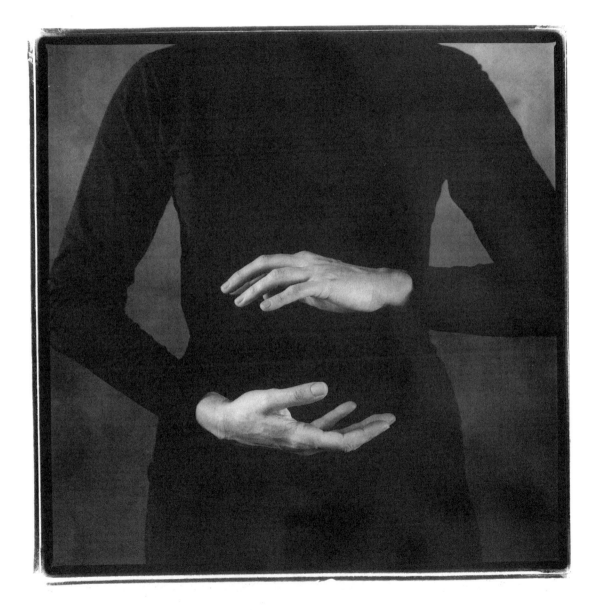

Pause Breathing

Pause Breathing is a technique for finding the natural rhythm you would express if no outside influences interfered. Once you feel your own relaxed rhythm, you have a comparison point for tension. Any time you want to regain a calmer sense of yourself, Pause Breathing helps you. Learn to do it lying down as described in the following exercise. Later you can use it any time, anywhere, as needed.

This exercise was developed by Magdalene Proskauer, a San Francisco therapist with a specialty in the psychological aspects of breathing. Her work uses breathing as a doorway to our dreams and a key to body alignment.

During an unusual crisis or an average routine, our breathing rhythms change with our moods. We tend to synchronize our breathing with the rhythms around us. If life's pace is too fast for comfort, slowing down our breathing promotes relaxation.

THE BASIC BREATH

Lie on your back on the bed or floor. Relax your arms at your sides and let your feet fall out to the sides. Close your eyes and feel the way you are lying on the floor. Notice whether any part of your body feels a bit tense or doesn't seem to be resting comfortably on the surface beneath you. Now move your focus inside your body and notice where you feel movement as you breathe.

If you feel tense anywhere, try imagining that you can breathe into the tension, as though you could actually exhale through that body part. Imagine the breath relaxing your sore muscle as it moves through it. Breathing into a body part is something you can do any-where, any time you feel tense or nervous. Locate the tight place and "breathe into it." Breathe in synch with the tensing (inhale) and relax-ing (exhale) of your movement.

As you are doing this exercise, loosen your clothing if it is tight at the waist. Let the muscles of your stomach and abdomen relax and let your breath sink lower in your body. Place one hand, palm down, at the lowest place on your torso where you can feel the motion of your breathing. Let your hand rest on this place a while until you begin to feel the rise and fall of your body under your palm from your breathing. Now let your hand and arm relax at your side again. If you see any pictures of yourself or other images during this breathing exercise, remember them and draw them or write them down later.

Relax your jaw and open your mouth a little so that you can exhale through your mouth. You don't need to breathe heavily. Relax and breathe naturally. Inhale through your nose; exhale through your mouth; and pause at the end of the exhalation before you breathe again.

This pause is the key to the effectiveness of the breathing. Crucial things are happening to your body during the pause; you are actually still exhaling, though you may feel as though nothing is going on. Deepening your exhalation gets all the stale air out of your lungs and makes more room for fresh air when you inhale. Most of us don't exhale deeply enough. Often, when you feel that you can't take in enough air, and that you'd like to inhale more deeply, it's because you haven't exhaled fully enough to make room in your lungs for new air. This is usually the breathing difficulty in asthma. Lengthening your exhalation can help release asthmatic symptoms.

You have paused at the end of the exhalation for a long time now. Let yourself really explore the pause. How does it feel to you? Does it feel too long? Not long enough? Are you a little worried that your body won't breathe in again unless you make it? Think of your breathing when you are asleep. You don't have to tell yourself to breathe then. Think of animals breathing when they are resting. Their breath is long and rolling. They don't tell themselves to breathe. You can learn to trust that your breath will always come in again.

Allow the pause to be as long as it wants. It may feel very long. See whether you can wait and stay with the pause until your body wants to breathe in again by itself. Inhale through your nose; exhale through your mouth; then pause and wait. It's a little like standing on the beach and waiting for another wave to come in. Try to find a pace at which you are neither holding your breath to prolong the pause nor making yourself breathe in again. Let yourself breathe in this pattern as long as you want.

What we call 'I' is just a swinging door
which moves when we inhale and we exhale.

—*Suzuki Roshi,* ***Zen Mind, Beginner's Mind***

II
RELAXING DAY TRIPS

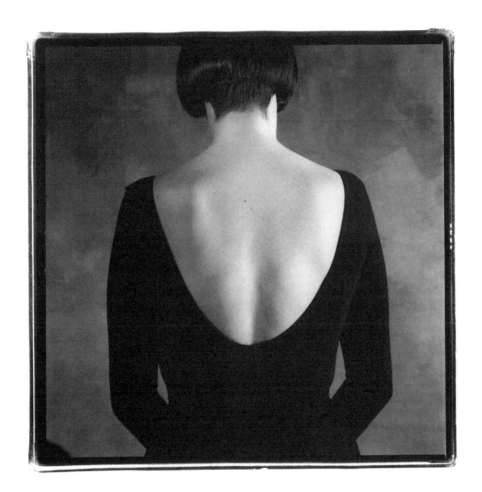

THE HIDDEN TREASURES IN PLEASURE

BUSY BACK CARE

HANDY TIPS

WEEKEND WARRIOR SPA

II

RELAXING DAY TRIPS

THE HIDDEN TREASURES IN PLEASURE

One thing I always knew how to do: enjoy life.
If I have any genius it is a genius for living.

—Errol Flynn, **My Wicked, Wicked Ways**

Being a chicken about pain turns out to be the better part of bodybuilding. Having survived the "go for the burn" exercise phase, we hear current health experts report what hedonists always believed: pain is the body's signal to do something else that feels better.

The sensation you have when you go for the burn in exercise is not primarily from melting fat but from muscles and tissues tearing. Because these tears take time to repair, you will progress more steadily toward your fitness goal if you push yourself up to but not past your pain limit.

The exercises in this section can be used to reduce daily aches and pains. They will also relax your back, neck, and other high-stress areas that can benefit from preventive care. If what you do is fun, you'll produce healthier results and probably do it more often. So go ahead. Enjoy yourself. The more pleasure the better. It's good for you. Raise your pleasure quota and increase your daily dose of joy. Doctor's orders.

Life is much too important to be taken seriously.

—Oscar Wilde, **Lady Windermere's Fan**

SHOULDER LIFT

Exaggerate and release.

1. Inhale as you lift both shoulders up as high as you can and hold this position for a few breaths. Exaggerating a tension pattern like high shoulders can help you become more aware of the condition and begin to notice when you are tensing.

2. Release your shoulder muscles as you exhale and allow them to sink as low as possible without pushing. Make your movements very slow and very smooth. You may start with jerky movement that feels as though your muscles are walking down steps. As you release your muscle tension, your motion will become more graceful.

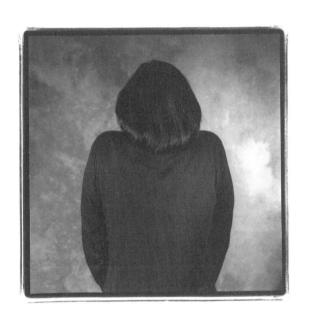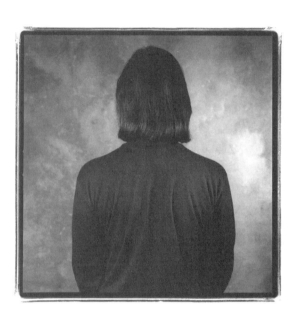

BACK BALL

Sphere pleasure.

1. Sit in a chair with support for your lower back. Hold an air-filled ball about six inches in diameter. Make note of the position of your back in the chair so you can compare it with your back angle after the exercise. Where is your back touching the chair?

2. Place the ball under the spine so you are wholly or partly sitting on it. Move until you feel comfortable. Then rest there a while and imagine you can exhale down your spine and into the ball.

3. Now remove the ball and sit on the chair again. Compare your back's position to when you started. Are different parts of your lower back touching the seat than when you began? Do you feel more cradled by the chair? Having a small lift at the base of your spine helps align your vertebrae so you can sit upright without straining. Use a small pillow when you don't have a ball.

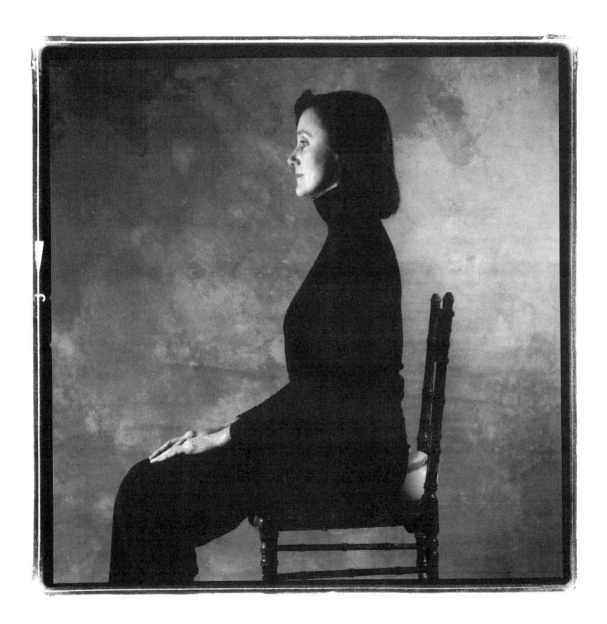

PENGUIN

▅▅▅▅

Become unflappable.

1. Hug yourself by placing your palms as close to the tips of your shoulders as is comfortable.

2. Press in hard with both palms as you press outward away from the spine with both shoulder blades. Keep your spine straight and your chin tucked under so you are lengthening your spine as you open your upper back.

3. Pivot at the waist from left to right and back so you relax your waist and rib area.

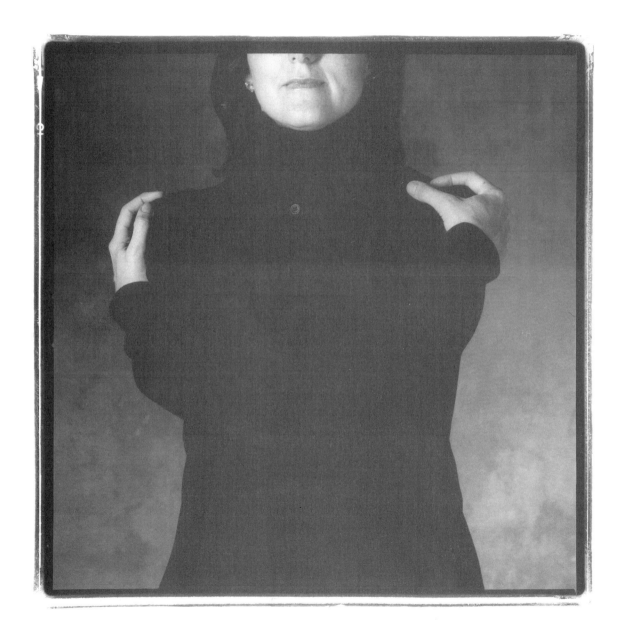

HALF PENGUIN

Wing it.

1. With one arm at your side, grasp the shoulder with your other palm. Stand straight and tuck your chin under.

2. Allowing your straight arm to hang as loosely as possible, pivot at the waist, pulling your shoulder from right to left with your grasping hand. Relax your shoulder and arm muscles as you turn.

3. Reverse and repeat the exercise on the other side. You will notice that one arm is markedly more relaxed than the other. See how loose your hanging arm can be in the shoulder socket and at the elbow and wrist.

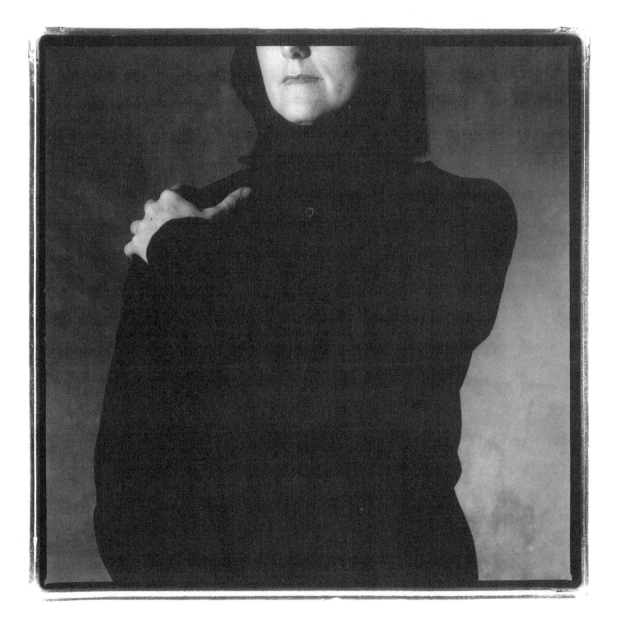

SEATED TOES TOUCH

Cross-pressing.

1. Bending forward at the waist, relax your torso onto your thighs and your head between your knees.

2. Place your right palm on your right foot. Inhale and cross your left hand over your right. Press down on the floor with the heel of your left hand. You will feel a stretch in your left upper back and ribs as you press. Hold this position and breathe deeply. Occasionally press down with your right hand also to intensify the back stretch.

3. Reverse your hand position and repeat this stretch for the right side of your back. When done, sit up slowly.

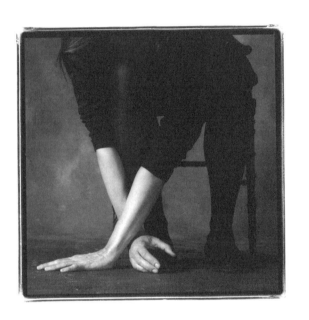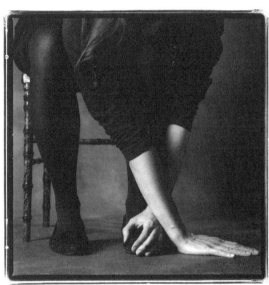

LAP REST

■■■

Lying in your own lap.

1. Begin by inhaling. With your spine straight, bend at the waist and lean forward over your legs. Exhale as you release your back muscles and rest your torso as close to your thighs as is comfortable.

2. Allow your arms to droop at your sides. Relax your neck and shoulders. From time to time turn your head from side to side to release your upper back. Breathe deeply without forcing it.

3. Close your eyes and imagine you can send your breath to different body parts to release any tension. Allow your lap to support your weight.

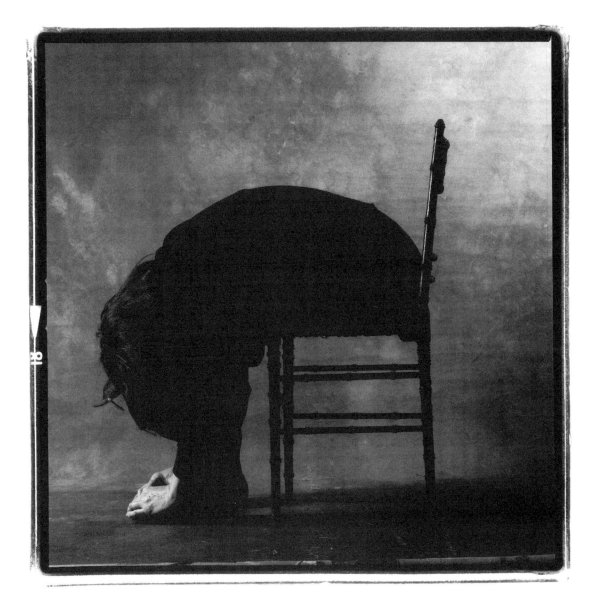

BUSY BACK CARE

Things on the whole are much faster in America;
people don't stand for election, they run for office.

—Jessica Mitford

Psychologically, the back represents our relationship to our burdens. Overburden or overwork frequently leads to back pain. Back care can prevent stresses from becoming back aches. A back rub for a tired friend can be a significant comfort.

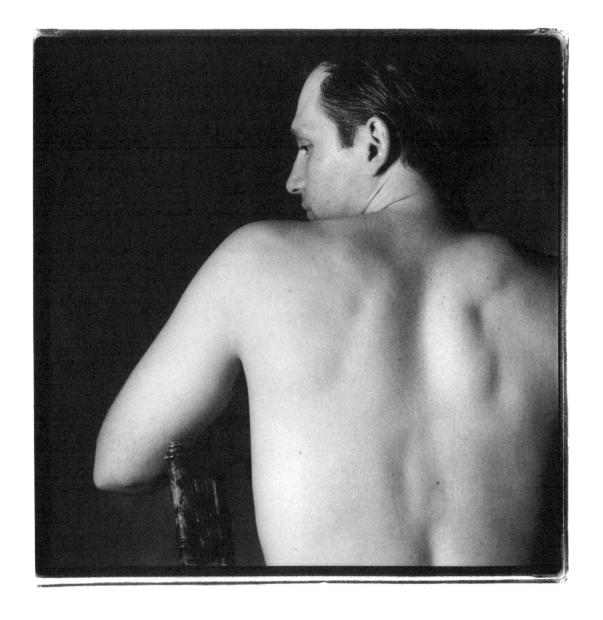

HONCHO HUNCH

Desk work.

1. Stand with your back to a stable chair or desk about hip height. Place your weight on the heels of both hands as they rest on the edge of the desk.

2. With your feet planted apart, exhale as you lower your torso and bend your knees. Sink until you feel a good stretch in your upper back. Hold this for several breaths.

3. On an inhalation, straighten your knees and stand up.

4. Lean your weight back onto your hands as you press forward with your hips to arch your lower back. At the same time arch your neck back and try to relax your head over the desk or chair.

5. Repeat this arch and hunch sequence in slow motion several times.

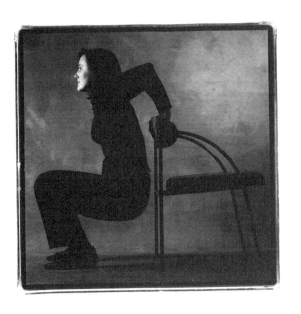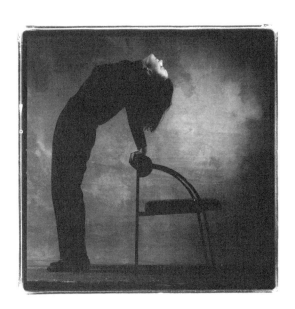

SPINE SQUAT

█████

A cracker.

1. Squat with your hands on your knees and your shoulders hunched so your weight is resting there.

2. Twist one shoulder toward the other while keeping your spine straight and your torso upright and forward. Exaggerate the twist to stretch all the vertebrae in your back.

3. Reverse and repeat to the other side. With practice you can crack your spine during this exercise. This helps relieve compressed areas along your spine. Try different angles in your twist and get leverage by pushing down with your hands. Stay as upright as possible for the best twist.

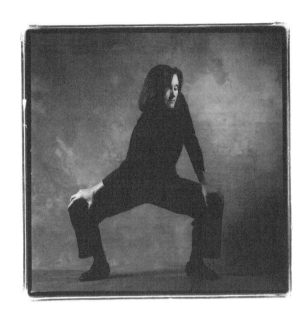

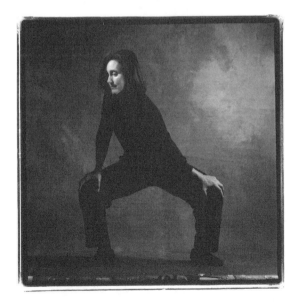

STANDING SHOULDER STRETCH

███

Reverse reach.

1. Place your right foot forward. Lean your torso over the leg as you stretch your clasped arms behind you.

2. Stretch your left leg out behind you and try to keep both heels on the floor. Relax your neck.

3. Much of the stretch comes from the position of your arms. See if you can reach your arms up so they are almost parallel to the wall.

4. Lower your arms slowly. Reverse leg positions and repeat on the other leg.

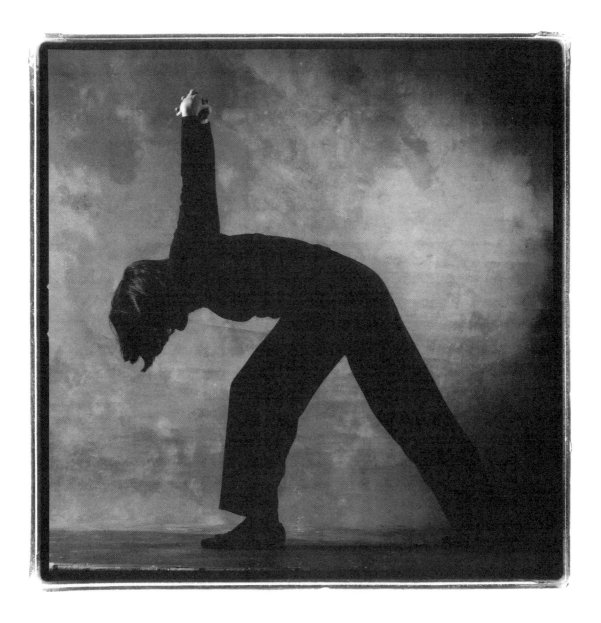

CORNER PRESS

Relax on edge.

1. Turn a corner into a back easer. Line the wall corner up with either length of muscle on either side of the spine. Do not press on the vertebrae. Lean back, pressing with your feet, to achieve pressure on a tight muscle.

2. You can press on one spot. Or you can try to flatten your whole back against the corner for a long massage. You can also move the massage from top to bottom of your spine as you roll your back against the wall.

3. Don't forget the other side of the spine.

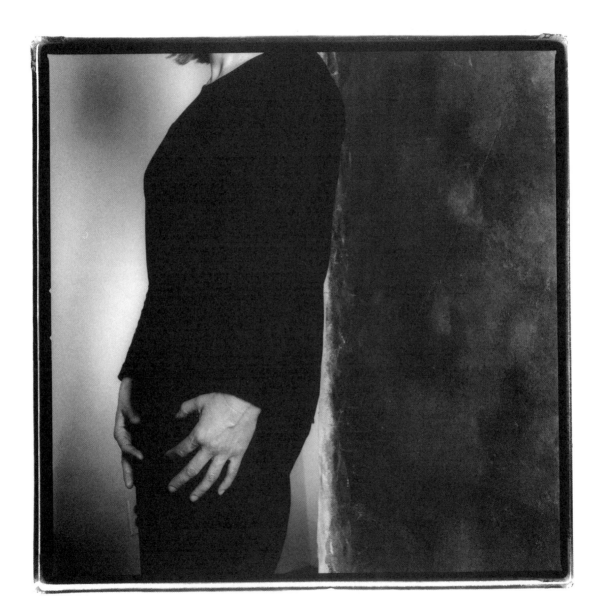

HANDY TIPS

*Do all work as if you had a thousand years to live
and as if you were to die tomorrow.*

—Ann Lee, founder of the Shakers

Hands represent our activities, our compulsions, and our sense of social distance. Relaxing the hands can ease our sense of anxiety at being overscheduled and overactive. A hand massage to a loved one is a sign of respect.

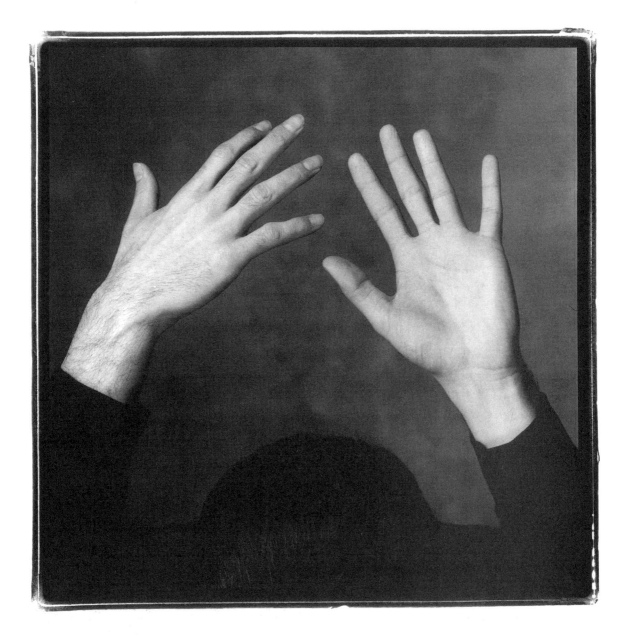

HAND POINTS

Massage these acupressure points on the hand for relaxation.

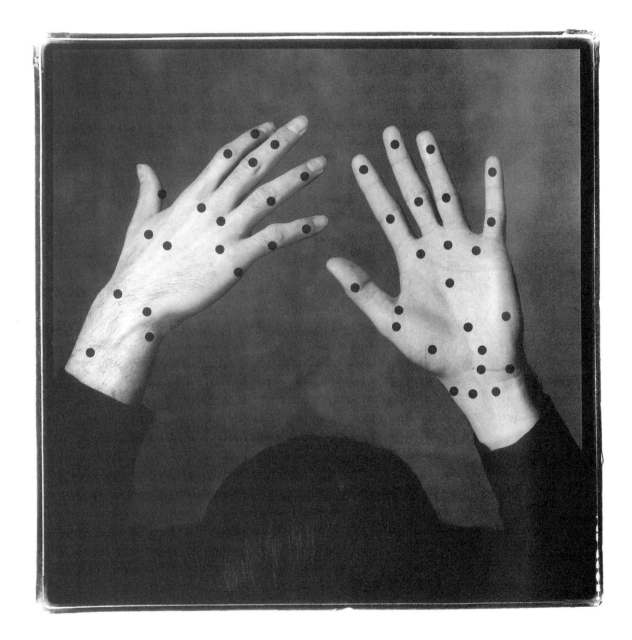

HAND PINCH

▬

A pinch can be an ounce of prevention.

1. Held in a pincer position, your thumb and forefinger form a fine massage tool for small areas. Slide them from the base of the wrist down the web of skin between each finger.

2. This massages the sensitive nerves between the bones of the hand. The thumb web has a specially powerful acupressure area.

3. For a final treat, pinch harder just as you briskly slide your fingers off the hand.

4. Continue this massage on the points shown in the hand chart.

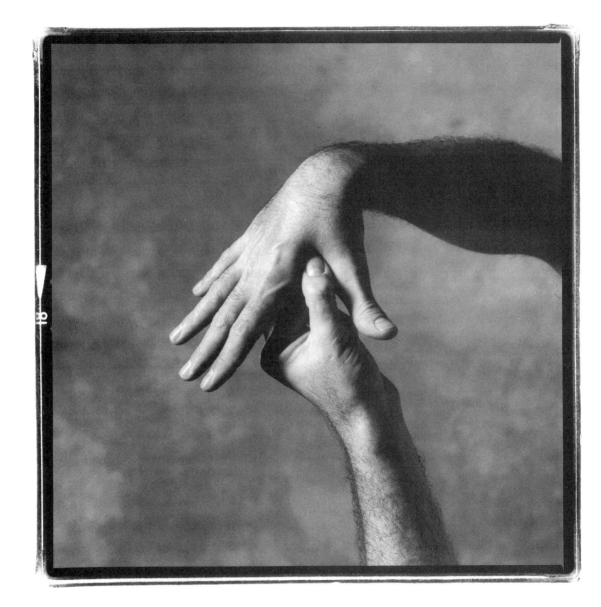

HALF BASKET

■

Half a basket is better than none.

1. When you'd like a thorough hand massage, but your favorite partner isn't nearby to do the Basket stroke (described in *Vacations for Two*), here's a way to do some detail work on your own. Interlock your fingers, but instead of twiddling your thumbs, use them to massage the opposite palms, pressing between the bones.

2. Spread the hand being massaged out taut. Use the fingers of your other hand to press upward behind your knuckles as you bend the fingers back as far as is comfortable on the open hand. This position will expose the sensitive area at the base of the fingers to be massaged. Feels best done with lotion or oil.

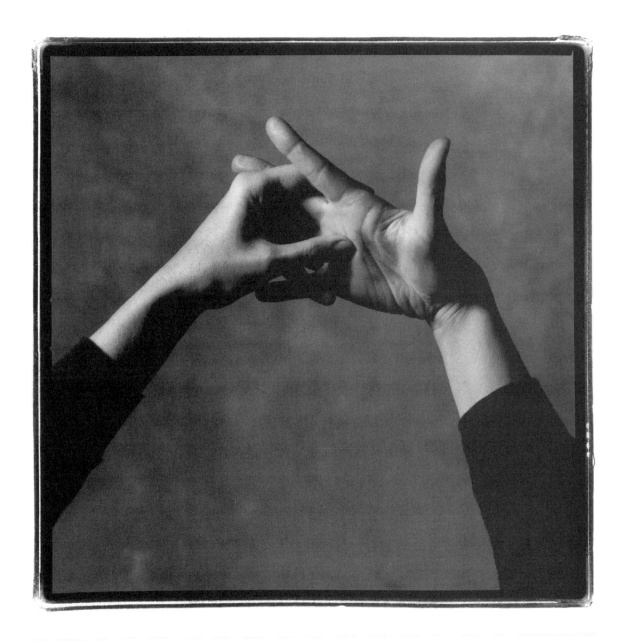

PALM FIST

Instead of pounding the desk with your fist,
use it to massage your palm.

1. Slide your knuckles over the palm, pressing deeply in between the bones. Oil or cream on the palm makes this stroke feel even better.

2. Try large circles on the palm with your flat fist.

3. Now switch hands and massage the other palm. Take your time and explore the structure.

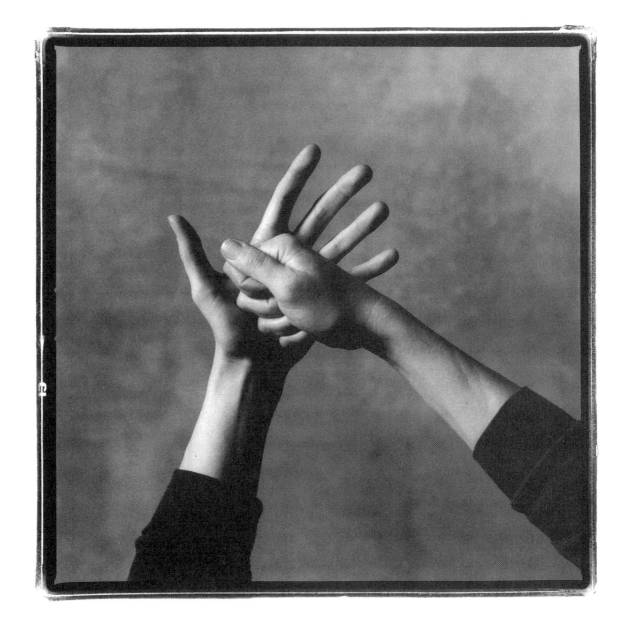

FINGER WRING

███

Feel like wringing your hands?
Add oil to make it relaxing.

1. Grasp one finger between your thumb and forefinger. Keep a steady pressure as you pull straight out toward the fingertip.

2. When you're about to slide off, quicken your pace so that the sensitive nerves receive an extra tug as you exit.

3. Return to the base of the same finger and try this variation. Spiral your fist in a corkscrew motion as you slide from base to tip.

4. Repeat on all fingers, using firm pressure and varying speeds.

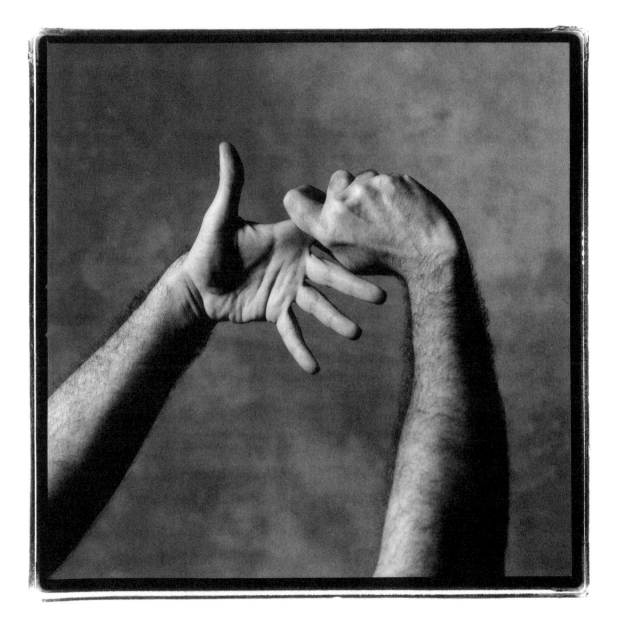

WRIST CIRCLES

■

Wring your wrist. (Not a neck.)

1. Without oil, grasp one wrist with the other hand and move the skin over the bone in circles without sliding at all. Repeat on other wrist. Work down the arm a few inches.

2. With oil, grasp the wrist and slide your clasped hand around the whole wrist at the same time as you rotate the circled wrist in the opposite direction as far as is comfortable. Repeat these opposing circles several times on each wrist.

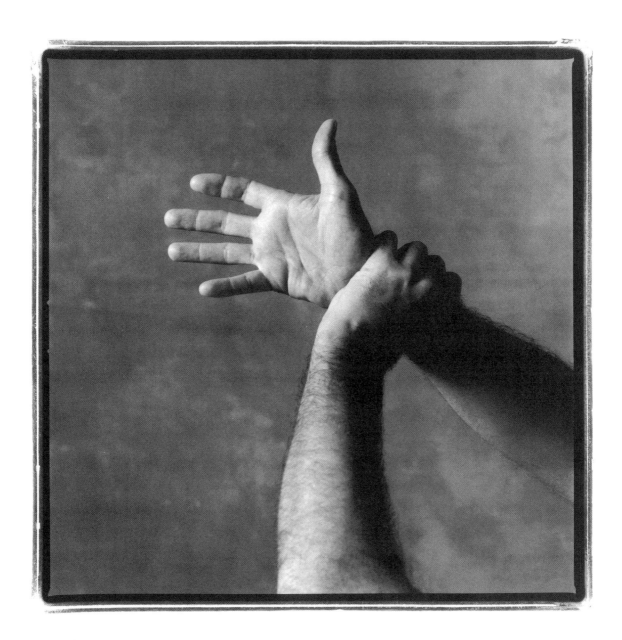

WEEKEND WARRIOR SPA

'Know thyself.' It is a difficult task, seductive and painful.
—Isabelle Eberhardt, **The Diaries**

Sometimes one makes mistakes.
—Greta Garbo *(on getting a permanent wave)*

After a week of relatively sedentary work, many of us overcompensate with strenuous weekend exercise. Noble as the impulse may be, it often leads to sprains and strains of unused muscles. The techniques in this section focus on areas most often bruised by Weekend Warriors.

No matter what shape you are in, any new activity uses new muscles. Impatience is not a virtue during physical exertion. Learn to listen to your own body language and respect your limits. Stretching before and after exercise is important to warm up and cool down. The following self-massage exercises lead you through a brief sports muscle treatment session.

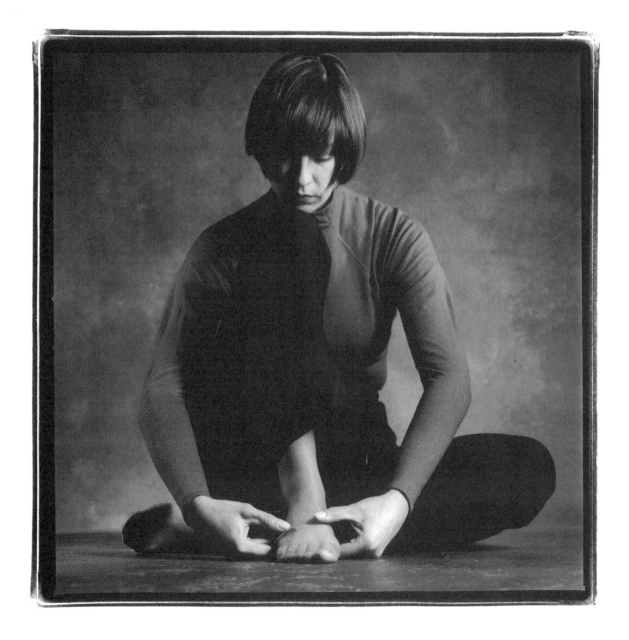

THIGH POINTS

The thighs have it.

1. Sore thigh muscles often result from strenuous exertion after long periods of inactivity. You can release tension in the area by massaging tight spots all over the top of the thigh.

2. Press in gradually and make firm circles on the area. As your muscles relax, you can press more deeply.

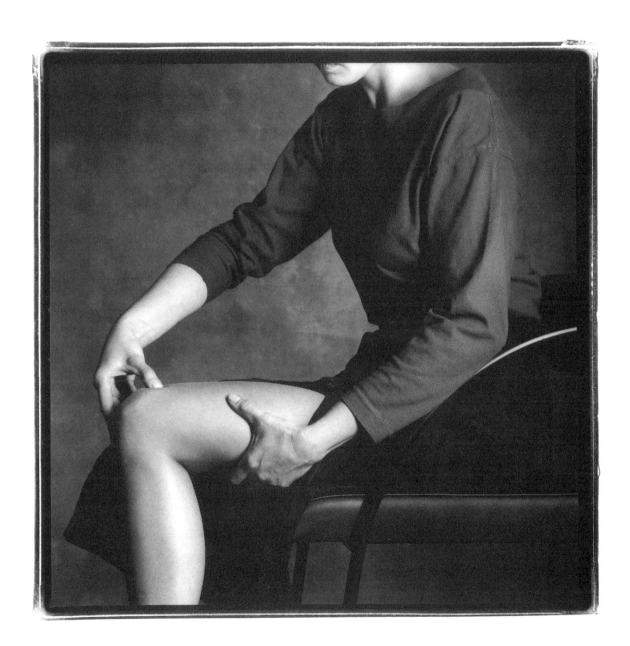

CHEST POINTS

Aid for a bruised ego.

1. If you have exercised strenuously and discovered you've over-stepped your capacity, you may be feeling silly as well as sore. Revive your spirits with massage on the chest, the body part associated with the ego.

2. Lightly rest your fists on your chest and press deeply with both thumbs. Massage in between the ribs and around the collarbones in small circles. Be thorough.

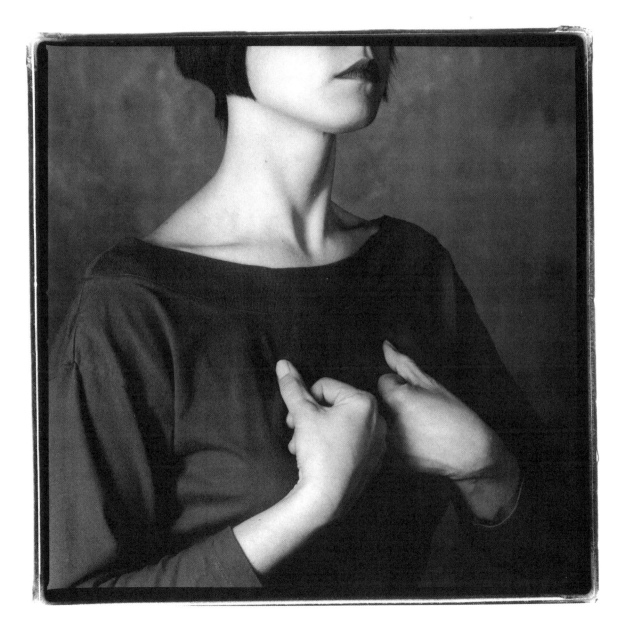

ARM MUSCLE ROLLS

Twist and sigh.

1. A gentle lift and rotation of a tense muscle can release a cramp or tight area. Relax the sore arm at your side.

2. Grab as much of the arm muscle as you can in your other hand and rotate it as far to the other side of the bone as it will go. Hold this position and breathe easily.

3. Then lighten your grasp and rotate the muscle back to its original position very slowly. You can use this muscle rotation anywhere you feel tense.

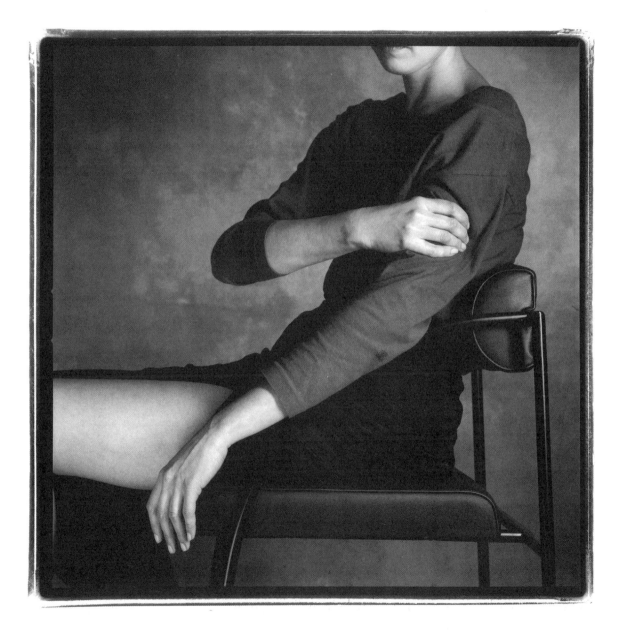

THIGH SLIDE

Pain push offs.

1. The long muscles of the thighs work hard all day and deserve some special release. Using your clothing as a sliding surface, make overlapping strokes from midthigh to the knee.

2. Lift your fingertips so the heels of your hands do most of the massaging. Try different speeds and pressures. Pay special attention to the six inches just above the knee, where much tension builds. Keep the motion continuous so it feels as though you are rolling an object along the muscle.

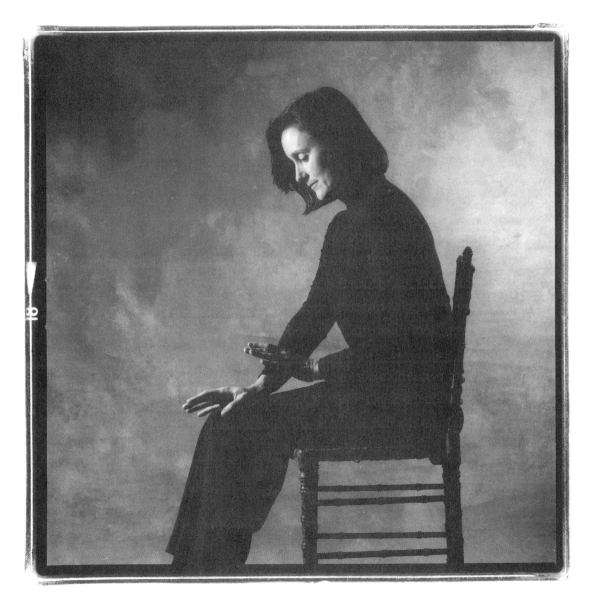

BACK BRIDGE—COW

▬

First you moo.

1. This hatha-yoga exercise is one of the most effective releases for lower-back pain and compression. Begin on your hands and knees. Inhale.

2. Drop your waist toward the floor as you press your hips up toward the ceiling, and tilt your head back, trying to look up at the ceiling.

3. This charming pose is called the Cow.

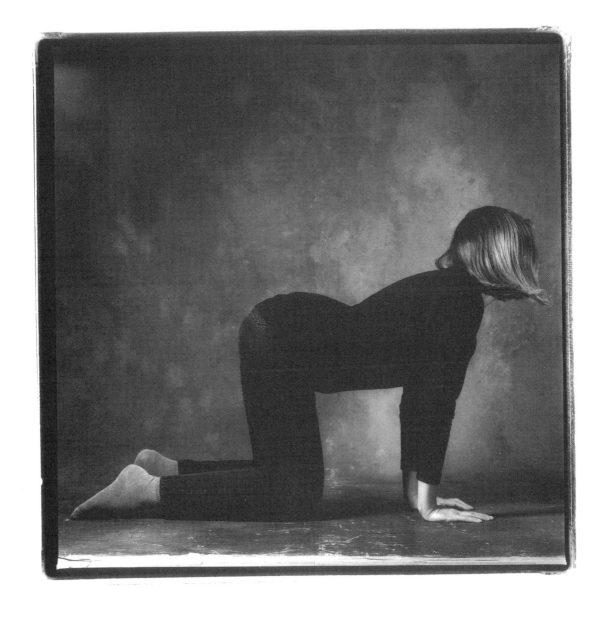

BACK BRIDGE—CAT

███████

Then meow.

1. As you start to exhale, lower your head, pushing your chin toward your chest.

2. Simultaneously tuck your pelvis under so that your back arches up toward the ceiling like a Halloween cat's.

3. Begin the Cow pose on your next inhalation. Alternate cow and cat positions with your breathing so that the motion is continuous.

4. Repeat this sequence several times a day if your back is aching. It is also an effective preventive exercise for daily back care.

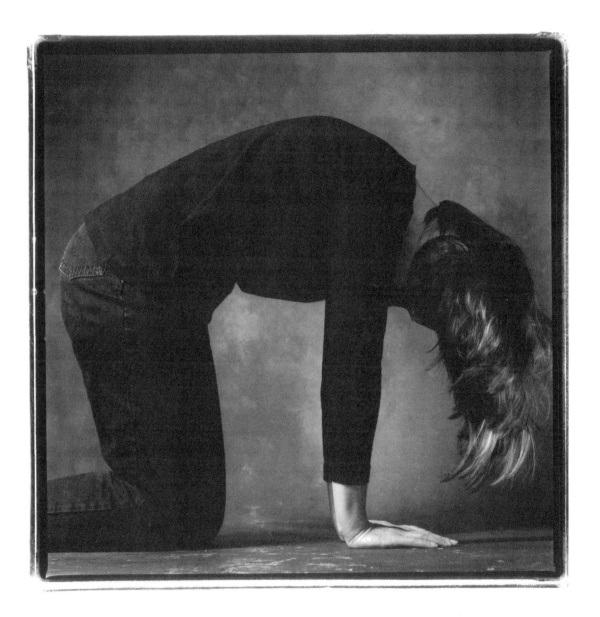

BIRD REST

Fold up for five.

1. This is a particularly comfortable position for a tight back. It is essentially a kneeling fetal position that can relieve spinal pressure.

2. Place your forehead on the floor and your arms resting at your sides. Inhale as you pull your shoulder blades toward each other and raise your shoulders off the ground.

3. Exhale as you ease the lift and lower your arms again. With each exhalation allow your shoulders to come closer to resting on the ground. A fitting finale to a hard week or weekend.

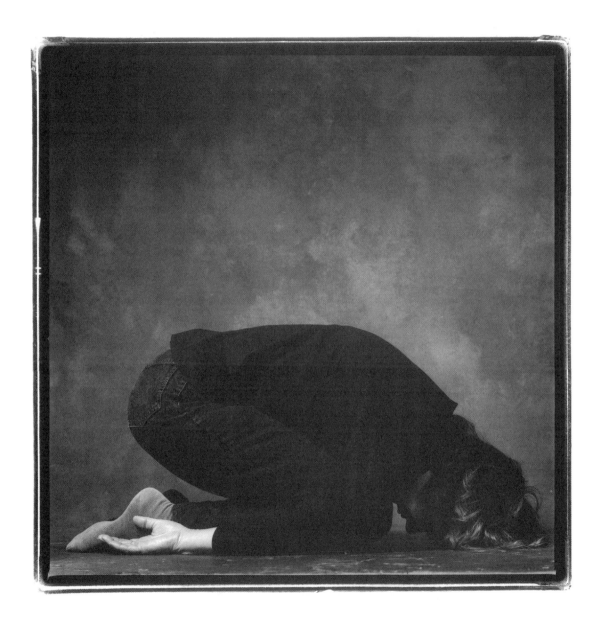

III
NIGHT FLIGHTS

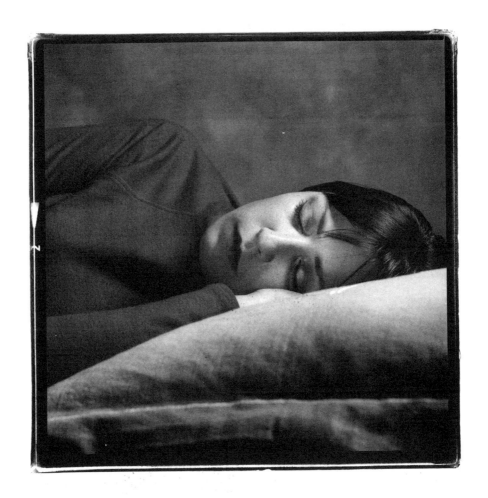

SLEEP CYCLES
SLEEPY ALL OVER
BACK IN BED

III

NIGHT FLIGHTS

SLEEP CYCLES

O gentle sleep, Nature's soft nurse!
—*William Shakespeare,* **Henry IV, Part II**

The day's journey into night can be made more satisfying when we learn about our body's natural sleep cycles.

Each of us needs about eight hours of uninterrupted sleep per night to maintain tiptop health. Every bodily function replenishes itself during sleep. Too little sleep produces a state of stress that weakens our resistance to illness because our disease-fighting systems have been deprived of the resting time they need to rebuild.

SMART NAPS

Timing is the key to a satisfying sleep. Naps are most effective when limited to thirty minutes or less. Many people notice that long naps can make them feel more tired than refreshed. This is because REM or deep sleep sets in soon after you pass the half-hour mark. Waking from the lighter sleep state of a short nap is much less of a struggle than from deep sleep. Even a half-hour rest gives your body time to partly revive its systems.

Your Cycles

Most of us have noticed that at certain times of the day or evening we consistently feel tired. Human metabolism cycles in hour-and-a-half intervals. To calculate your personal sleepy and alert cycles, start counting from one of your obvious tired times. For example, if you tend to become drowsy at 10 P.M. each night, your next sleepy cycle will climax at 11:30 P.M., then 1 A.M., and so on. The peaks of your waking cycles also come at hour-and-a-half intervals. They start forty-five minutes after your sleepy cycle. Don't bother trying to fall asleep at 10:45. If your sleepy cycle started at 10, you won't be really tired again until 11:30.

Knowing your cycles will also help with morning plans. Set your alarm for the height of your waking cycle rather than your sleepy cycle. Remember: More sleep will not make you feel more rested if it means you have to get up during the next sleepy cycle.

The exercises in this section are designed to slow down your metabolism and can be done in bed to relax muscles often cramped at the end of the day. You can do them while waiting for your next sleepy cycle. Sweet dreams.

EYE PALMING

Don't peek for five minutes.

1. The eyes work hard all day and need revitalization to avoid strain. You can do this standing up or lying down.

2. Cup both palms over your closed eyes. Relax your neck and arms and remain in this position for as long as is comfortable.

3. Visualize that you are sending your breath on each exhalation down your arms and into your palms to revive your tired eyes.

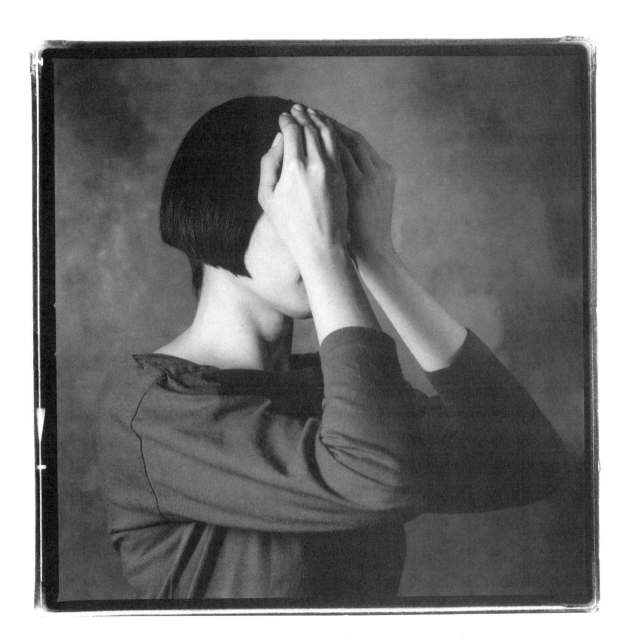

SCALP POINTS

▬▬▬

Top priority.

1. There are powerful acupressure points and nerves all over the scalp. When things come to a head at home or office, don't lose yours. Massage it. Start at the top and make your way thoroughly down the sides and the back of the head to the base of the skull.

2. A particularly relaxing technique for scalp points starts with light pressure on a fixed spot. Stay put on one area as you increase finger pressure. When you have reached your desired pressure, move the skin of the scalp over the bone by rotating the fingers without sliding at all.

3. Then lift the hands and find another area to massage and repeat this rotation-in-place technique.

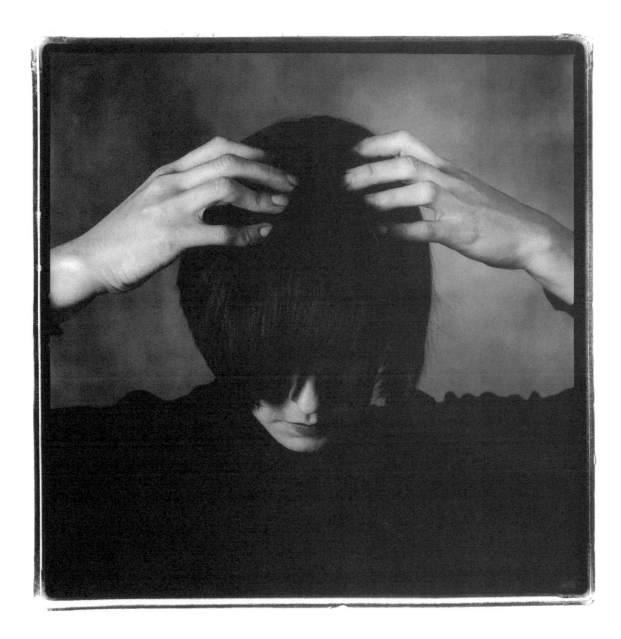

SLEEPY FEET

Feet first.

1. Massaging the feet sends relaxation throughout the body as you rub the foot's nerve endings, which connect with other parts of the body. When you're too exhausted to exert yourself much, foot massage gives maximum results for a minimum of effort.

2. Roll onto one side and rest your upper knee on a pillow to prevent back strain. Draw your knee high enough on the bed so you can reach your foot with your upper hand, and use it to press around your ankle and over the bottom of your foot.

3. If you're still awake, roll over and repeat on the other foot.

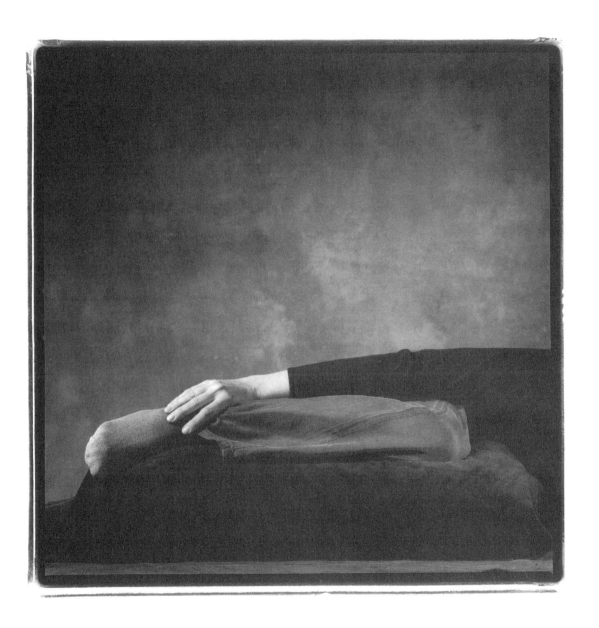

H I P   F E E T

■

The hipbone's connected to the knee bone.

1. Many people injure themselves while they are resting.
Holding one position for a long time taxes the muscles. So if
you sleep in a position that twists or puts pressure on your body
in stressful ways, you can develop cramps or even pull your back,
hips, or neck out of alignment. Sleeping with your knees higher
than your hips relieves back pressure.

2. Try placing a pillow or rolled towel under your knees as you
lie on your back. If you can sleep this way with your head fairly
flat on the bed, your back and hip joints will experience the
least pressure.

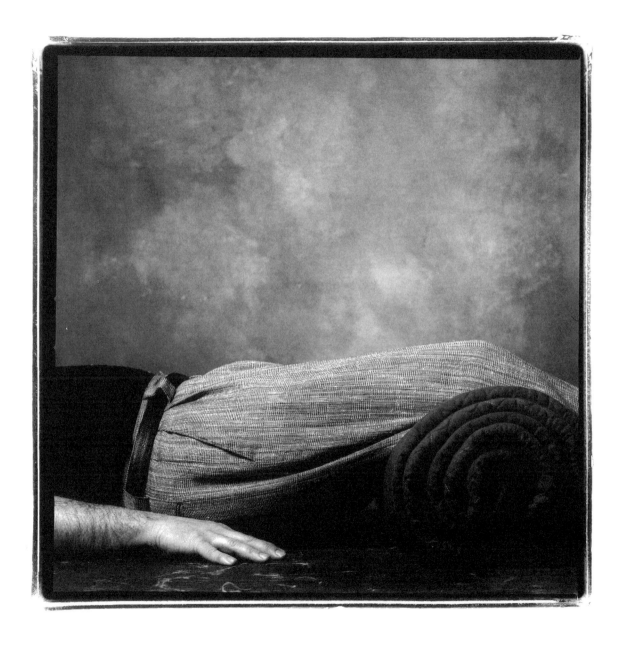

BED BALL—NECK

Have a ball relaxing your neck.

1. This is one of the most relaxing treatments for a tired or sore neck. Lie down on your back with your knees elevated by a pillow. Place an air-filled rubber ball about six inches in diameter under your neck. Find a place for the ball that allows you to give over the work of holding up your head completely to the ball.

2. The more you allow the ball rather than your neck muscles to hold your head, the more aligned the vertebrae in your neck will become. Imagine that each time you exhale, you can send your breath into your neck muscles to relax them from the inside.

3. You can also roll your head slightly from side to side over the ball as you inhale and exhale to massage your neck muscles.

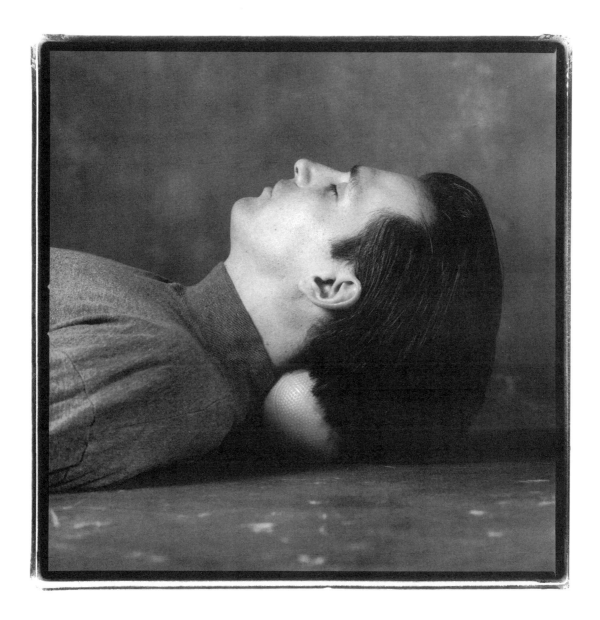

BED BALL—LOWER BACK

■

Backs relax around balls.

1. A six-inch ball filled with air can give a great massage to your lower back. Lie on your back with the ball under the base of your spine. Move the ball around until you find a place where your back feels completely comfortable when you put your weight on it.

2. As you exhale, imagine that you can breathe down through the center of your spine and into the ball. With each breath, let your muscles relax more.

3. The tilt given by the ball and the flexibility of an air-filled ball allow your lower back muscles to release.

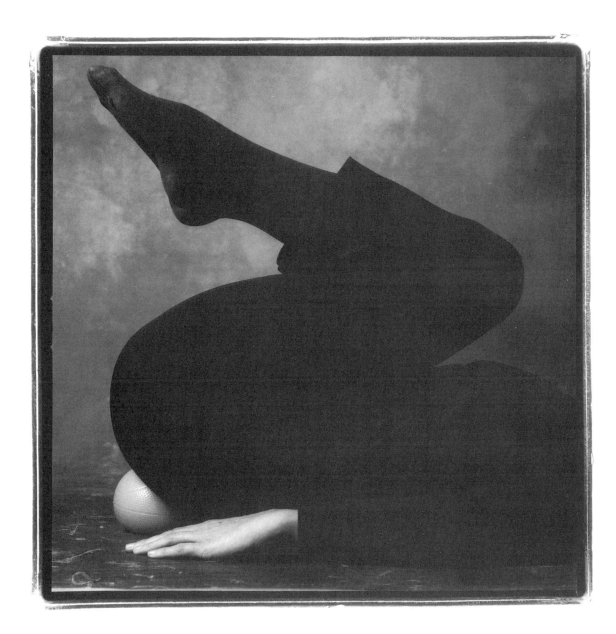

SWAN FOLD

A graceful bow.

1. Add an arm motion to this exercise. As you roll your head to the left, roll your arms to that side also. Try to make the arm and head movements smooth, slow, and continuous.

2. Try rolling your head in an opposite direction from your hands for a different upper-back relaxation.

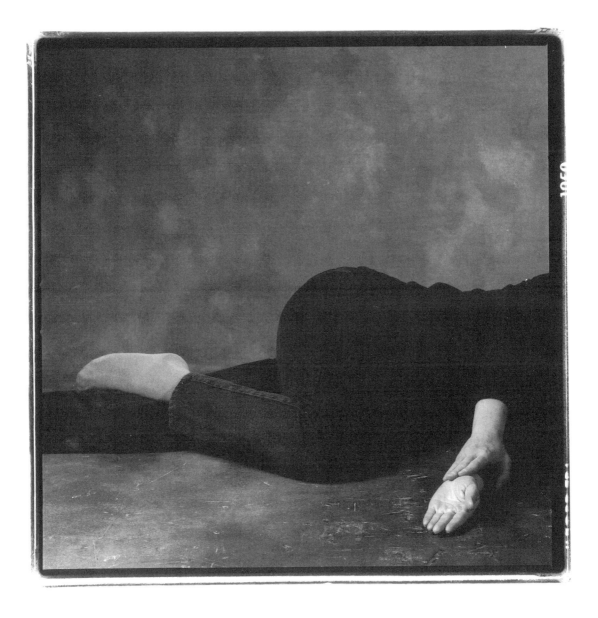

KNUCKLE PRESS

Knuckle down.

1. Downward pressure on the base of the spine can leave your back aching. Before you go to sleep, relax your lower back with some massage. If you are tired, you can use your body weight for pressure by lying down on your knuckles.

2. Bend your knees and place the knuckles of both clenched fists under the base of your spine. Just lie there and allow your body weight to sink more and more onto your hands. The coccyx bone at the base of the spine is arrow shaped. Angle your knuckles to fit on top of this bone to either side of the spine.

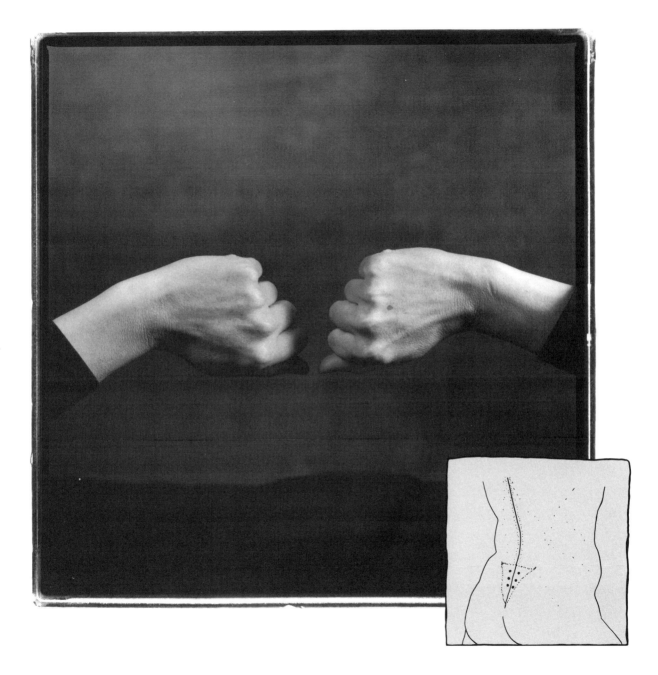

TWIST AND RUB

For sleepy backs.

1. Lying on your back, fold one bended knee over the other leg kept straight.

2. With the palm and fingers of your upper hand, massage any sore or tight areas of your lower back.

3. You can rock your hips back toward your hand from time to time to create more pressure.

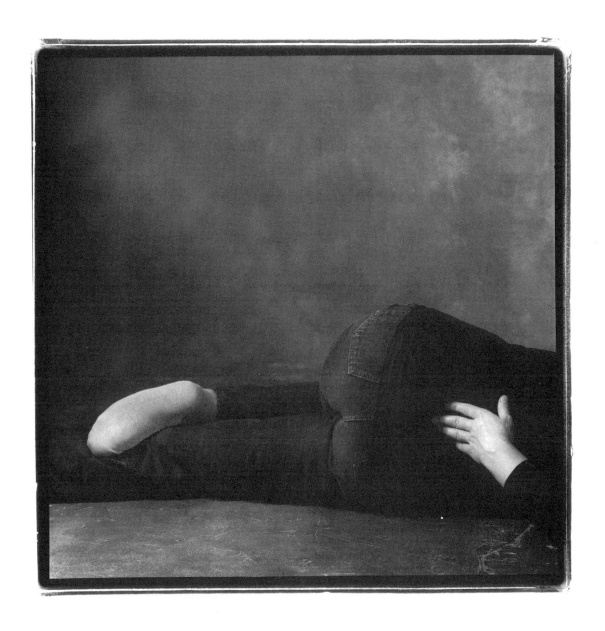

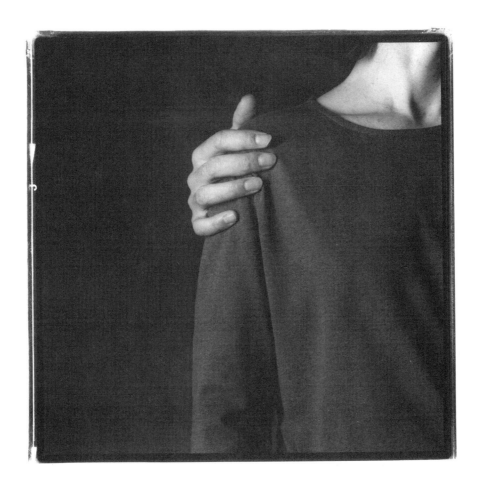

TICKETS FOR TWO
RELAXING PARTNERSHIPS
BACK TO BACK

VACATIONS FOR TWO

TICKETS FOR TWO

All day long they depend on each other,
without being dependent on each other.

—Tozan, **Zen Mind, Beginner's Mind**

Most of us know how to relax by ourselves, but staying calm and balanced in the presence of others is another matter. Someone you love can throw you off center as easily as someone you loathe. The impulse to lose track of ourselves and focus on the needs of another can confuse us in both miserable and happy situations.

The exercises in this section can help you become aware of your patterns in response to people and events that excite, frighten, or anger you. Use the breathing to return to your own body rhythm when you feel off-center in public. No one will notice you're doing it, so it can be useful in the middle of a crisis when you want to calm down, get back in touch with your thoughts, and focus. The couple exercises help you understand how you interact. They also feel good, are fun to share, and can be helpful tools when both of you are out of sorts and need to relax. Happy trails.

RELAXING PARTNERSHIPS

Usually, without being aware of it, we try to change something other than ourselves, we try to order things outside us. . . . When you do things in the right way, at the right time, everything else will be organized.

—Suzuki Roshi, ***Zen Mind, Beginner's Mind***

HEAD LIFT

Give it up.

1. The head is surprisingly heavy and requires constant effort during the day to keep upright. Having your head lifted and moved by a friend can be a pleasant relief.

2. Place both palms under the head, where you secure a firm, supportive grasp. Watch your friend's muscles and slowly raise the head on the next exhalation.

3. As your partner gives support of her head over to your hands, try moving the head slightly to one side and then the other, then up and down.

4. When having your head lifted, the more you allow a friend to move the head, the more relaxed your neck muscles will become. When ready, slowly lower the head to the ground.

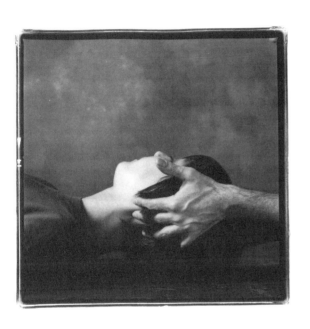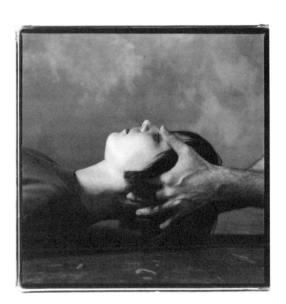

CHEST LIFT

Trust me.

1. This can be very relaxing for the neck and upper back. Lie down on the floor on your back. Reach up and give your hands to your partner.

2. As the partner, grasp your friend's wrists firmly. On her next exhalation, slowly raise her back and shoulders off the ground. Plant your feet to either side of her pelvis.

3. Encourage your partner to release the holding in her neck and let her head hang loose backward. Slightly rock her shoulders back and forth by pulling one toward you while letting the other go.

4. When you're ready, ease your partner *slowly* to the floor. Place the head down very gently.

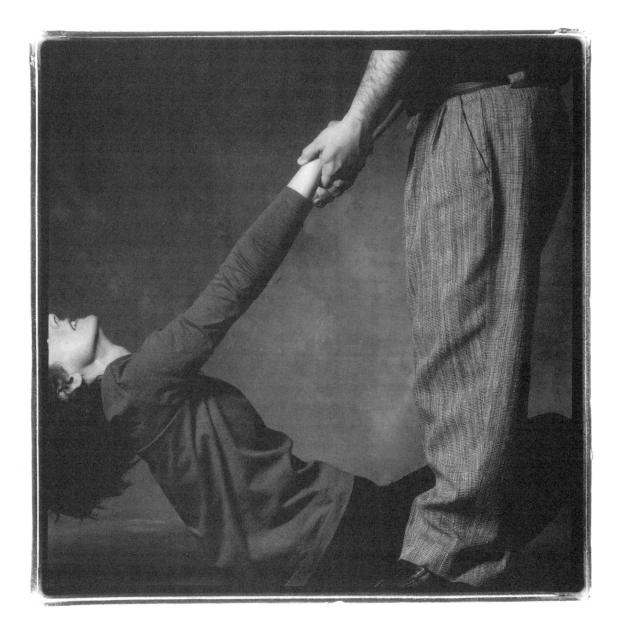

ARM LIFT

Hold on.

1. The arms rarely receive special attention; however, they do accumulate much tension from daily activity. Lifting and moving the arms for your partner can release the tight arm muscles.

2. Support the elbow in one palm and the hand in the other. Keep the elbow bent. Slowly lift the arm and make circles in the air so that the shoulder is rotated smoothly.

3. If you are receiving the lift, try to allow your partner to do all the work of moving your arm. When you feel muscle resistance, imagine you can exhale into the muscle.

4. After several circles, lower the arm softly. Repeat on the other arm. Be careful to move only in natural directions so the arm is not strained.

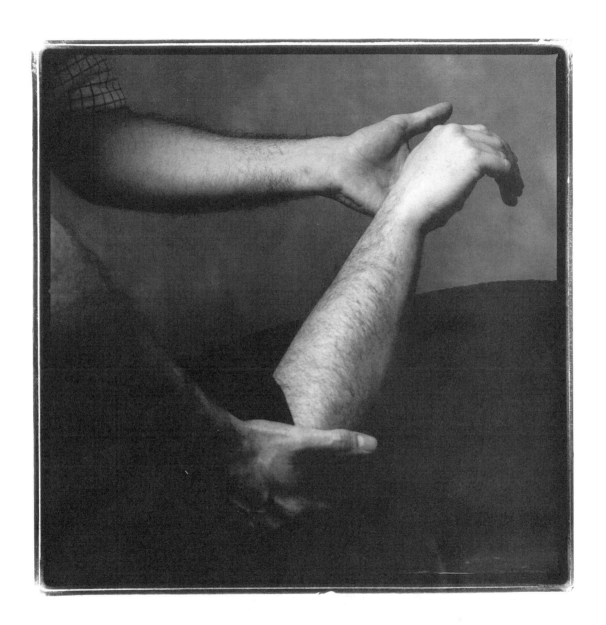

PALM BASKET

Give a friend a special hand.

1. This stroke sounds more complicated than it is. Once you've had it done, you'll know it's well worth the effort. Be sure to massage in between the bones at the base of each finger. These crevices are rarely touched, and pressure here feels delicious. Position your fingers as follows. Courage.

2. Place the little finger of your left hand between your friend's forefinger and middle finger; the fourth and middle fingers of your left hand between the forefinger and thumb; and the forefinger of your left hand on the other side of the thumb.

3. That was only the left hand. Now for the right. Place your little finger between your friend's middle and fourth fingers; your fourth right finger between the fourth and little fingers; and your middle and forefinger on the other side of the little finger.

4. In position, press down with your thumbs and up with your fingers so that your friend's palm is taut and the fingers are slightly arched back. Now use your thumbs to methodically massage the tiny grooves between the bones of the hand. This feels best with oil or lotion on the palm.

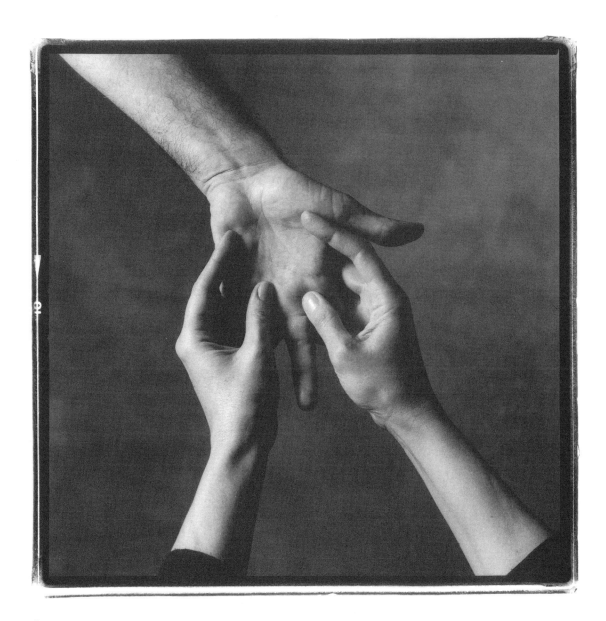

ELBOW PRESS

▅

Put your elbow on my shoulder.

1. Your partner should be sitting comfortably in a chair with his head relaxed forward.

2. Bring the heels of your hands up to your chin and place your elbows on either side of the base of your partner's neck. The large muscles stretching across the top of the shoulders are the trapezius muscles, which can become very tense from stress. Very slowly lean your weight onto your elbows.

3. Apply more weight only when you feel the muscles soften slightly, a sign of relaxation. When you are ready to release, do so gradually.

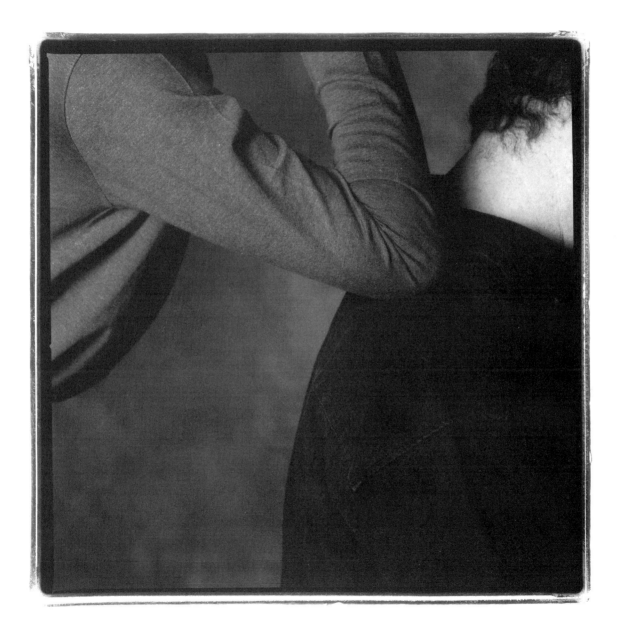

LEG LIFT

Teach an old muscle a new trick.

1. Stand near your partner's feet as she lies on the floor on her back. Grasp one ankle or arch with one hand as you hold the knee from underneath with the other hand. Your partner should try to release her muscles and let you do all the work as you bend the knee and raise the foreleg off the floor.

2. Then slowly move the leg, making circles in the air with the knee, and moving the knee as close to the chest as it will go without resistance.

3. At any resistance point, simply change directions and move a new way. The more your partner allows you to do the moving, the more her muscles will release any tension they might have accumulated.

4. Lower the leg slowly. Repeat with the other leg.

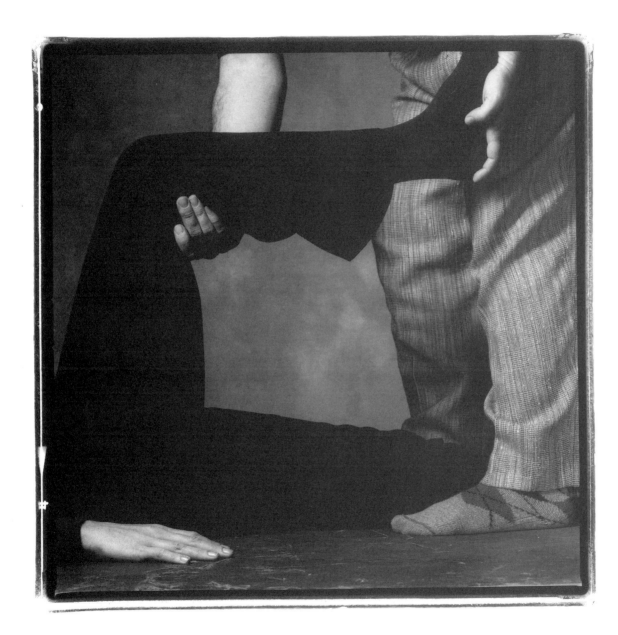

BOTH FEET TREAT

Relaxing squared.

1. If massaging one foot is good, massaging both is even better. Your partner should lie or sit comfortably so that her back and legs are well supported. Place one of your hands on each of your partner's feet.

2. Massage both feet, pressing deeply with your thumbs all over the bottoms of the feet and the ankles and toes.

3. Synchronize your hand movements so that the hands are both doing the same thing at the same time, and move rhythmically.

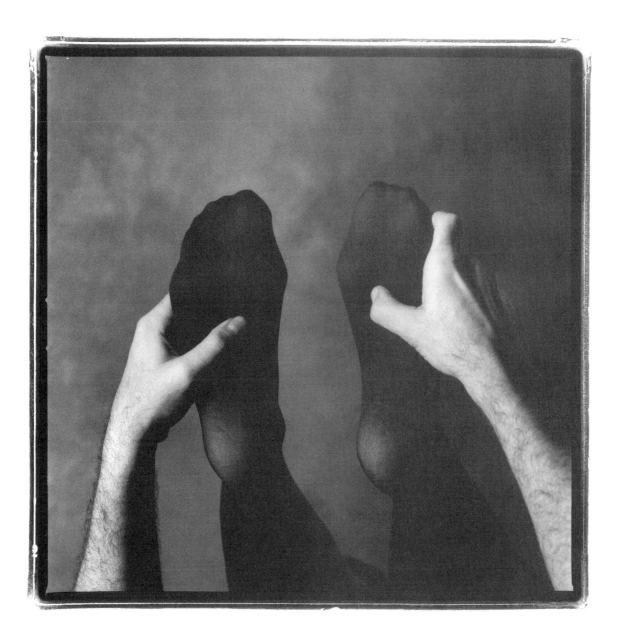

THE ROCKING HORSE—
ROCKING BACK

Lean and lose tension.

1. Sit opposite your partner on a rug or mat. Place the soles of your feet flat against your partner's. Hold hands together and spread your legs and feet as wide apart as is comfortable.

2. Inhale and lean back, giving your weight over to your partner's hands. Your partner leans forward as you lean backward. Relax your neck backward.

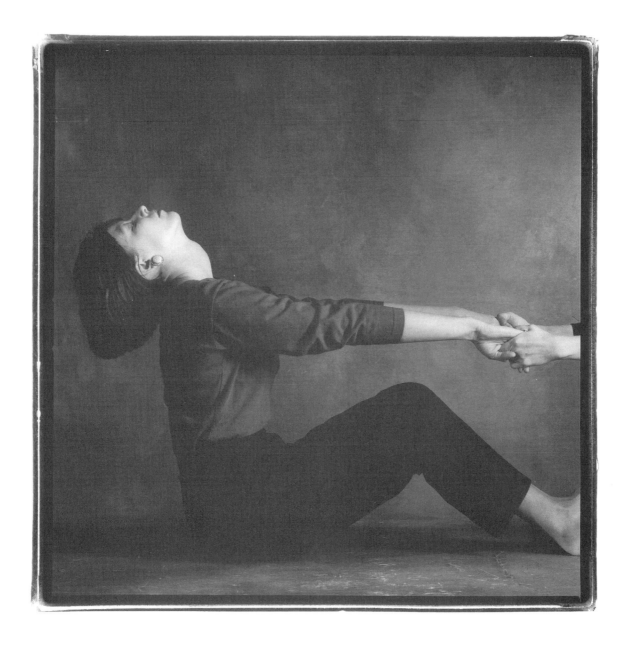

THE ROCKING HORSE— ROCKING FORWARD

A seated back stretch.

3. As you exhale, lean forward as far as is comfortable over your legs.

4. As you lean forward, your partner leans backward, and vice versa. Develop a rhythm so that the movements are smooth as though you two were on a rocking horse. Relax your back and leg muscles more each time you lean. Try to allow your partner the stretch she needs to reach her comfortable limit.

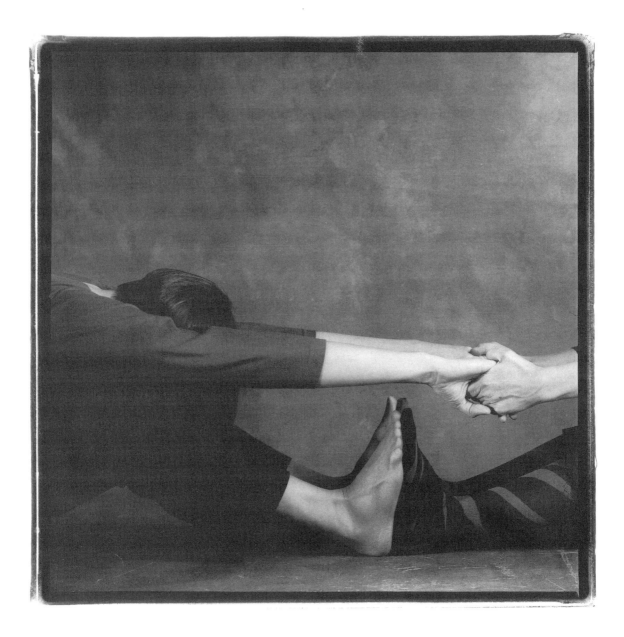

FOOT TRADE

■■■■

Foot friends.

1. Sit at either end of a sofa in which your back is well supported. Find a comfortable position in which one of your feet can rest in your partner's lap, and one of his can rest in yours.

2. Massage the whole foot with both your hands. Be thorough. You can mirror image your partner's massage, or independently proceed with a different one.

3. Trade feet and massage the opposite one now.

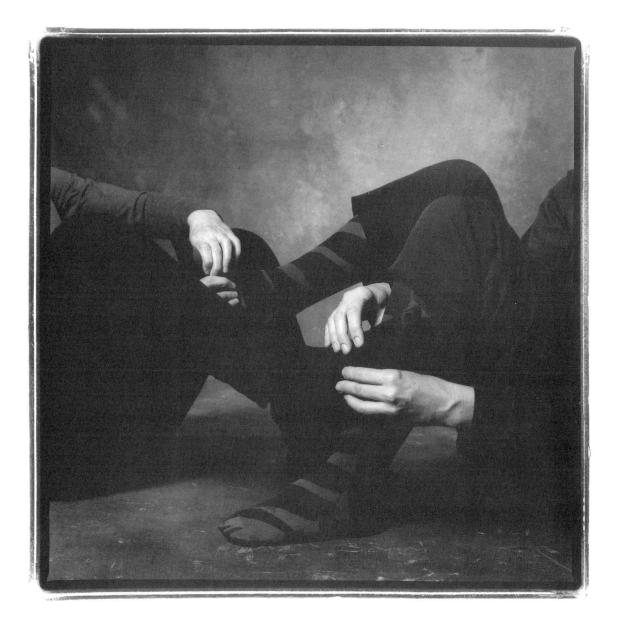

BACK TO BACK

BACK POINTS

To help relax the back, massage the muscles on either side
of the spine in the areas shown on the chart.

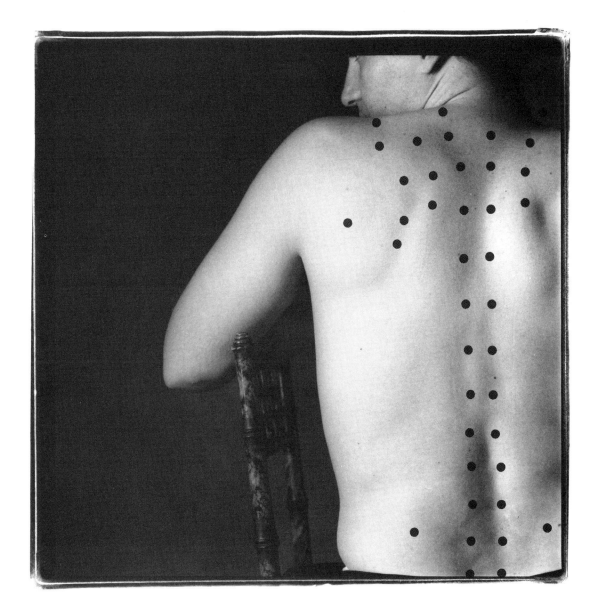

BACK-TO-BACK MEDITATION

Two breaths can be more relaxing than one.

1. This exercise can be a very relaxing meditation. If you take note of your back positions and your breathing rhythms, you can also learn subtle things about the relationship between your level of relaxation and your responses to other people.

2. Sit on the floor with your knees bent and your feet comfortably crossed. Relax your hands, palms up, on your knees. Sit back to back. Without talking, let your partner know in what position you are most comfortable so that neither of you feels too leaned on or leaning and your spines are touching as much as possible. Relax your breathing deep in your abdomen. Feel your back muscles move as a result of your breath.

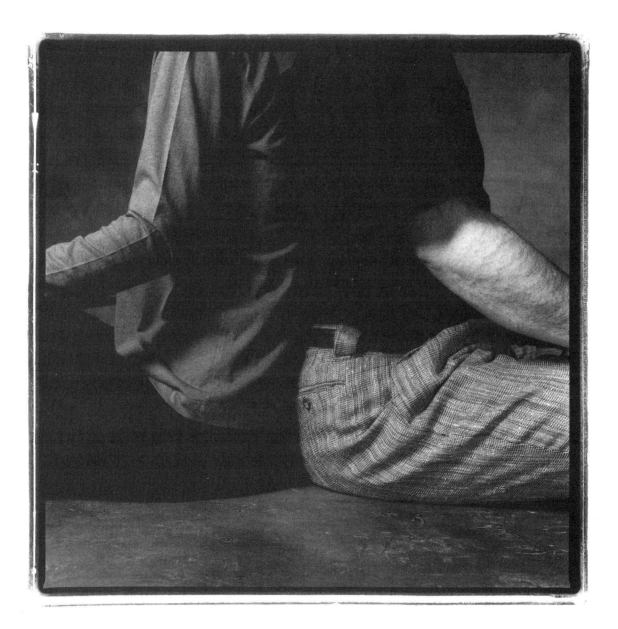

BACK-TO-BACK MEDITATION

An arm up.

3. Once you can feel your muscles moving in your belly and your back as a result of your breathing, try to tune in to your partner's breathing. Where can you feel the muscles moving from his breathing?

4. Notice whether you changed your breathing while searching for your partner's. Did your breath rise higher in your body? Did you synchronize your breath rhythm to your partner's without thinking? Most of us lose track of our own rhythms around other people and often take on their pace.

5. Relax your breath in your belly again. Can you feel your partner's rhythm without losing track of your own?

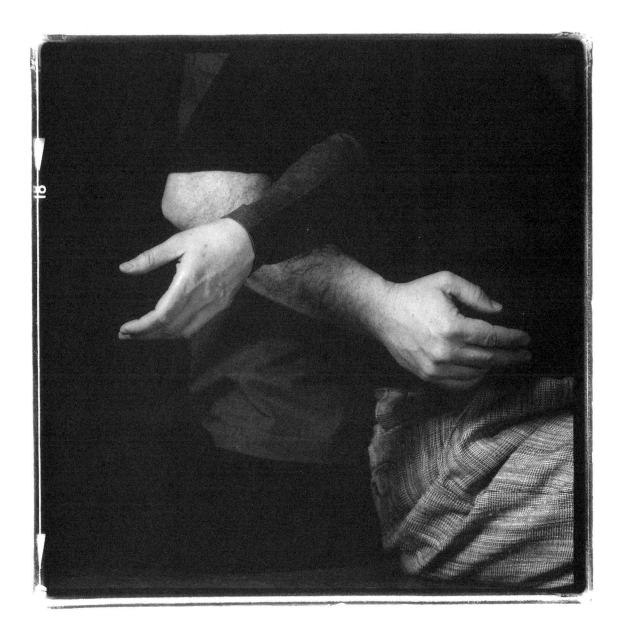

STANDING ON YOUR OWN FOUR FEET

Halfway there.

1. When you are ready, lock arms at the elbows. Bend your knees and bring your feet flat on the ground as close to your hips as you can.

2. Without talking, see if you can help each other stand up together by leaning on each other and pushing up with your feet. Success has nothing to do with muscle strength. It depends on how well the two of you can communicate nonverbally and balance your pressures. If the floor is not slippery and the two of you match your back pressure, you'll stand with ease.

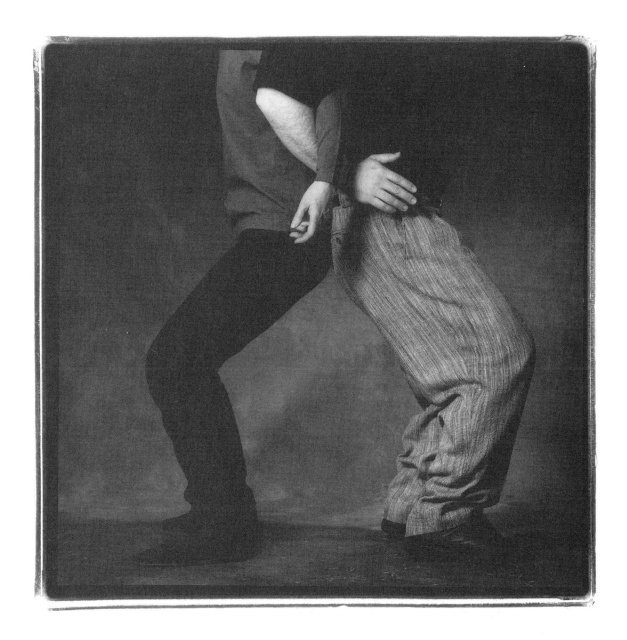

COCCYX PRESS

The arrow points down.

1. The coccyx, an arrow-shaped bone at the base of the spine, is crossed by many nerves leading away from the spine, down the lower back and legs. Massage here can release much back and leg tension.

2. Use your thumbs to press to either side of the spine on the muscles on the coccyx. Pressure and release should be very gradual. If you hold the pressure a while without moving your thumbs, this can be quite relaxing.

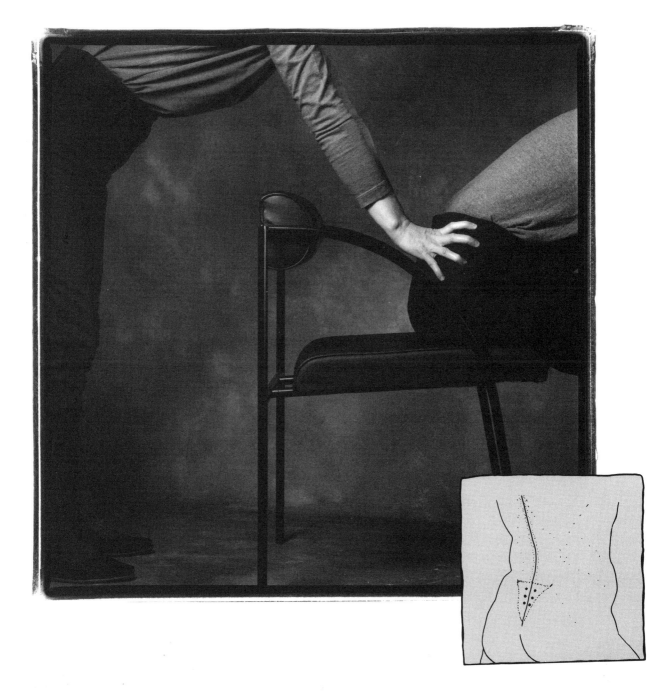

SPINAL PAT

This is spinal pat.

1. Your partner should be relaxed in a chair with her head on her arms on a desk or table. Use the taut palms of both your hands to apply light pats all over her back.

2. This technique feels best when it is applied systematically, shoulders to lower back and up again, for instance. Patting in a rhythm rather than randomly also enhances the relaxation.

3. Each person varies in the kind of pressure she prefers. Ask your partner if you should pat lightly or briskly.

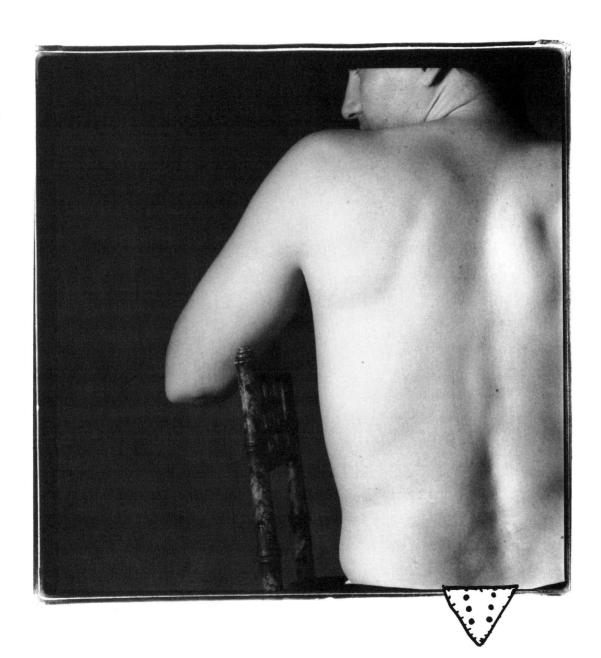

VERTEBRAE COUNTDOWN

The spinal frontier.

1. Starting at the base of the neck, place your thumbs on either side of the spine in the small grooves between the vertebrae. Never press directly on the vertebrae.

2. Gradually apply and then release pressure in this spot.

3. Then lift your thumbs and move them down the back to the next space between two vertebrae. Repeat the cycle of slow pressure and release. There are thirty-three vertebrae. Work methodically down the whole back. Each area will have a different degree of tension. Stay longer if tight. Take your time and be thorough and this massage will feel gloriously relaxing.

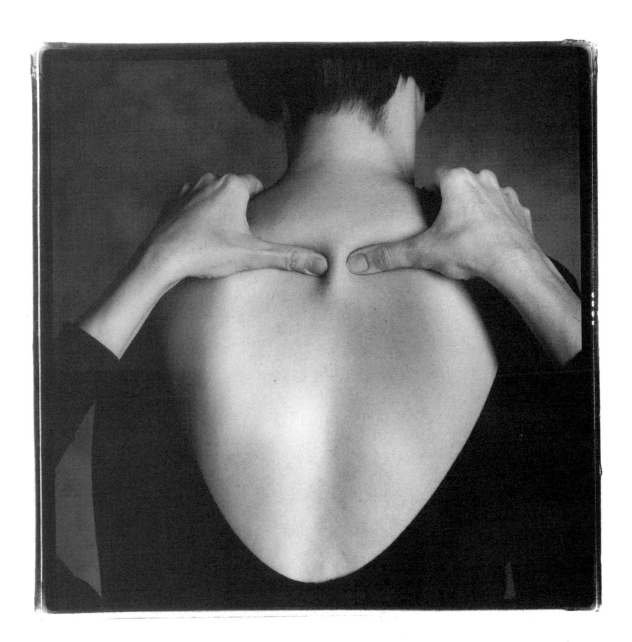

V

INDEX OF EXERCISES

INDEX

I do declare, you're the best kind of friend a body ever had!
—Scarlett O'Hara, **Gone With The Wind**

CREDITS AND
ACKNOWLEDGMENTS

Appreciation to the relaxed models:
>Marshall Stevens
>Dana Harbron
>Eugene Ruffalo
>Susan Orzal
>Anne Kent Rush
>Catherine Stone
>Jeff Stone

Orzal's hair by Marina, Monhair, New York.
Rush's hair by Tami, Barbara's, Fairhope.

Many thanks for special stress-reducing assistance from Freude Bartlett, Susie Glickman, Sandy and Eddie Levin, Ruth Morrison, Dawn Radtke, Peter Truce, T. Fang Wong, and Mu Shu.

ANNE KENT RUSH

Anne Kent Rush lives in a cottage on the shores of the
Gulf of Mexico, where she researches preventive health care
in the sun. Her books include: *The Back Rub Book* (Vintage);
Romantic Massage (Avon); *The Basic Back Book* (Summit); and
Getting Clear: Body Work for Women; Feminism as Therapy; Moon, Moon;
and *The Massage Book* (all Random House).

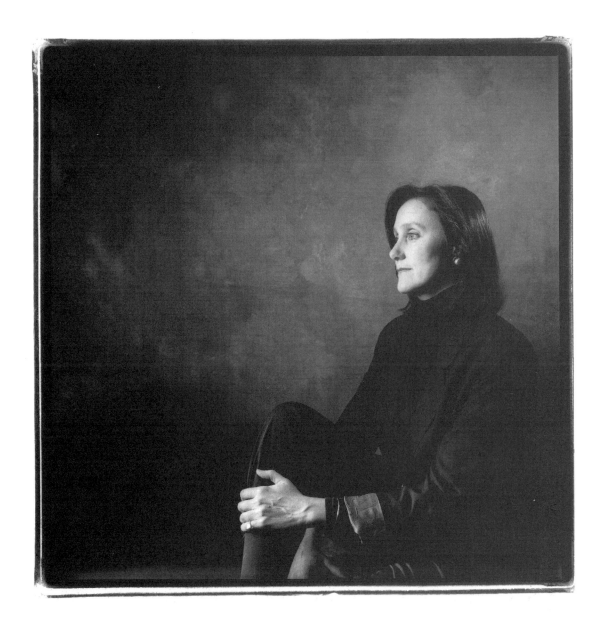

PATRICK HARBRON

For years, Patrick Harbron has been photographing people
for books, films, and magazines. His work has appeared in
*Newsweek, Time, Esquire, Rolling Stone, Premiere, The L.A. Times Magazine,
The New York Times Magazine,* and elsewhere. In film and TV,
Harbron has taken on assignments for Columbia, Disney, NBC,
and HBO, which have involved work with stars ranging from
Bette Midler to Arnold Schwarzenegger. In the music world he
has numerous album cover credits, and long experience working
with a variety of recording artists such as Bruce Springsteen,
Madonna, Hall & Oates, and Van Halen. Professional recognition
for his work has taken the form of awards from *Communication Arts,
American Photography,* and others. A native of Toronto, Harbron
currently lives in New York City with his wife Dana.

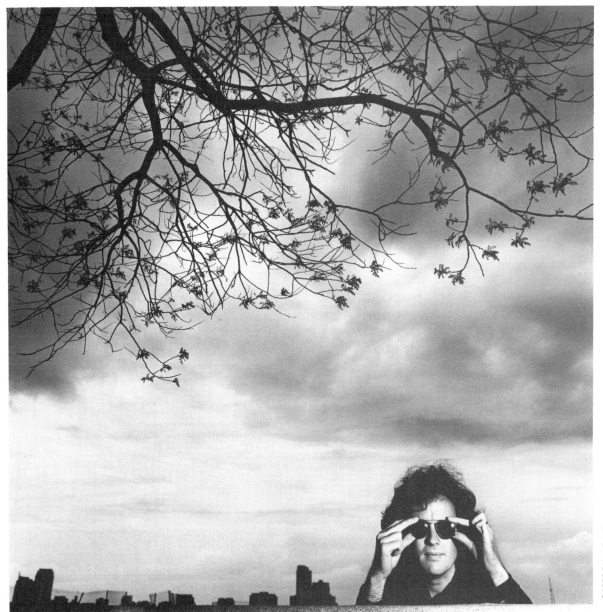